A Traveler's Guide to the Earth Experience

How to Pack Only What You Need

A Traveler's Guide to the Earth Experience

How to Pack Only What You Need

Kevin Poulston, DC

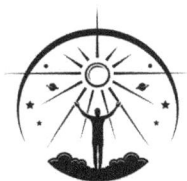

BEYOND BELIEF
PUBLISHING
—PUBLISHING—
YOU HOLD THE FUTURE IN YOUR HANDS

www.BeyondBeliefPublishing.com

This book is dedicated to one of the most amazing teachers that I have or will ever have—my mom, Bette. Without her, obviously, I would not be possible, and this amazing life experience would not be possible.

Contents

CHAPTER FIVE

Acknowledgments

I would like to express my gratitude to:

God, for being my creator, my savior, teacher, and mentor.

Mom, for being the most amazing tour guide through this life.

Pop, for his strength and unfailing support—you have always been a rock.

My brother Brian, for standing by me, for protecting me, and for giving me good advice.

Stacy, for showing me what it means to truly have an open heart.

Kim, not only for being one of my best friends, but also for helping me to put all the pieces together.

The publishing team at YouSpeakIt Books for the ease and grace of the process that brought this book into being.

Introduction

This book is about me and my experiences, but it was written for you. It was written for anyone who wants to make changes in their life.

As for me, I am doctor of chiropractic, with a specialty in energetic chiropractic. I balance cells through spiritual, mental, emotional, and physical parts by integrating them. I do this through a series of physical adjustments, emotional releases, and integration.

In my lifetime, I have worn many hats. I have an associate's degree in parks and recreation. I have written grants for children's programs, started a surfing contest, and have been a public speaker. I have lived in St. John in the Virgin Islands, Costa Rica, and England. But what I always *do* is help people. My passion in life is to help others.

So, the purpose of this book is simple: it was designed to help *you*.

I want to help you *take action*. Many of us want to change something about our lives, but we don't know how or where to begin—or if we should begin at all. Sometimes people become stuck in a fearful place, where they do nothing at all. It is a debilitating place to stay, and too many people stay there.

In this book, you will not find a guide on how to be a good spouse, or a good kid, or a good worker, although you may find ideas that can help you reach these goals. This book is simply an action guide that you can apply to your own life. It is a field manual for you, from which you will glean insights into how you can get moving toward your goals. If your life is not moving in the right direction, this book will help you figure it out.

Simply put, this book is designed to give you some recipes, if you will, that can help make your life better.

There is a real need for these simple recipes. With the current state of affairs in this country, I see so many people who are spinning around in circles, just hoping for the best.

I hear people say, "Oh, this next generation—they are walking around like zombies."

My counter to that is that I don't think this generation is any less capable than any other generation. However, many of us, especially the young adults of this generation, don't have the tools we need. Some of us weren't given any tools at all; others weren't given the right tools for life in today's world.

We need some guidelines. We need some direction. And, we need some hope.

I am hoping that this book provides a little of each of these things for you. Even if it helps you move only a single step forward, that's a step in the right direction.

You may be regretting mistakes you've made. One beautiful truth about life is that we all make mistakes. Great! Go ahead and make mistakes, but be sure to learn from them. Don't create your life out of a series of mistakes from birth until death.

You may be focused on achievements. Reaching achievements is good. However, if all you are doing is achieving, you might want to push yourself further—enough so that you make some mistakes. That is where growth comes from. It's the balance, guys and girls; it's the balance that is important. You can't have the good without the bad. You can't have the bad without the good. Savor all of it, the good and the bad.

People always ask the big question: *What is the meaning of life?*

There are two important facets to the answer: First, the meaning of life is your perception. We will discuss this further in the first chapter. The second distinction is one that has changed my life substantially. It is the understanding that this life experience is an emotional one; it is not an intellectual one. The meaning of life can't be found by thinking; you must experience it.

We are here to enjoy, savor, and experience all the different spices of life, all the emotions. Many people go too deep into their heads, myself included. Life, however, is not an intellectual experience. I don't mean that we don't use our brains; of course, we do. But the true meaning of all that is happening to you can't be found in your intellect.

I often hear people ask questions like: *Why is all this happening to me?*

What is happening in your life is exactly what you need to experience in order to grow—in order for your soul to grow.

Your life doesn't stay in a single station; it is constantly flowing, or moving. You are not meant to be stuck or running around in circles. If you rely on the brain to get you through this life experience, then you will miss the boat in many ways—you will miss out on *the whole,* the true purpose.

We all know someone who's filthy rich. They may have all the money in the world. They could have ten PhDs and be accomplished authors. However, some of these people have rather empty lives. If they have kids, their kids don't want anything to do with them. They might have been through a series of divorces and are lonely now. They may have a beautiful mansion up on the hill with a drawbridge, lakes, fields, and expensive toys. What they don't have is happiness.

It's not my contention that these are bad people. It's that they missed the whole purpose of why we are here. You must *feel* it. It is like sitting around in a nice restaurant having a nice piece of steak. Savor every bite.

When you are reading this book, I ask you to feel it with your heart. When you are going through the experiences of your life, feel them with your heart. Your brain will get you through to a certain level, but then it just can't take you any further.

Love is a good illustration of this concept. Love is one of those ideas that you can sit and think about, or write about, all day, without your heart ever feeling it. Your brain is not going to help you understand or experience love. You've got to feel it.

As you go through life, learn to ask yourself: *Does this feel right?*

If you ask yourself how it *feels* when you are wondering about an experience, you will instantly know the answer. Whether you listen to that answer or not—well, that is up to you—but when you ask yourself what you feel, you will instantly know, for certain: *This isn't good. This is bad. This is great.*

I encourage you, Reader, to feel this book rather than only using your brain. Use your heart. Certain things are going to hit you. Don't take my word for it, just read on and see for yourself. Pay attention, and see which ideas hit you in the heart.

You will have an inner sense of awareness when you come across one of these: *I don't know what he's talking about, but it feels right.*

When you have this sense, get ready for some sort of insight. It is during these moments that the magic can truly happen for you in your life, and new growth will begin. Keep this in mind while you are reading this book.

We all read to learn, and learning is a kind of growth. When you read, you are educating yourself. You are raising your vibration. There are a number of ways to look at this. In gaining more knowledge, you will be encountering new ideas, and you will raise your vibration. In short, you are enlightening yourself.

This is what I hope for you to gain from reading this book— new ideas—even just one new idea. One idea can change the world. It is another light bulb.

When Thomas Edison had this new idea for a light bulb, everyone called him crazy, but he kept working on it, through many failures.

When an associate visited Edison in his laboratory and attempted to sympathize with him regarding his lack of results, Edison responded: "Results! Why, man, I have gotten a lot of results! I know several thousand things that won't work."

Edison went through so many trials, and, even when it just wasn't working, he didn't quit. He recognized that every failure was a learning experience that could lead him forward.

You are traveling through life as I am, and sometimes, it can be a bumpy road. For the moment, it may be that—just like Edison—you are figuring out all the wrong ways to proceed.

That's fine, though, because you are learning many things along the way. Just like Edison, when you get one thing right along the way, it will propel you to the next level.

Above all, Reader, as you proceed from day to day, it is my hope that you find a greater sense of love for self—and that you extend this love to others as well. Learning how to treat others better while you struggle—while we all struggle—will come back to nourish your own heart and help you attain a true sense of joy and hopefulness in life.

CHAPTER ONE

Achieving Your Purpose-Driven Life

HOW TO BEGIN: TAKING INVENTORY

Before you embark on any journey, it's critical that you clearly see where your launching place is located.

Where are you starting out?

Let's say you are hiking the Appalachian Trail, and your goal is to hike fifteen miles. If you don't know where you're starting on that trail, you will never know when you hit fifteen miles, or surpass it. If you are setting off on your life-changing journey, you must know where you are, right now.

Take a personal inventory to help you visualize your starting place. This will also give you a way to check on your progress toward your goals. In making this inventory, you will also be setting your intentions—either consciously or subconsciously—and this is an important part of the process.

The Definition of Health: Spiritual, Mental, Emotional, and Physical

Your health has four different components.

- Spiritual
- Mental
- Emotional
- Physical

These are the four equal parts of health, and all of them are essential to your well-being.

How well do you understand these four parts?

Most of us have a good idea of at least one, two, or maybe three parts, but it is rare for any person to fully understand all four of them. You cannot actively strive for true health until you can put all four parts into the picture.

Let's look at each of them more closely, so we can understand them better.

Spiritual

What is your spiritual understanding of the world?

A spiritual element can be anything from mind to God. Your spirituality doesn't necessarily have to include God—it may include Buddha, or karma, or another spiritual force—but something *outside* of yourself is essential for spiritual health.

If you are setting yourself as the entire center of the universe, that is a heavy load to bear. The weight of the world will be on your shoulders, so to speak. Spiritual health is having something outside of yourself to turn to when the stuff is really hitting the fan.

Mental and Emotional

The mental and emotional parts of health are often thought of as linked together, and it is true that they are closely linked. However, there is a difference. A mental reaction can simply be an opinion that you have on something, without any emotional content. For example, you can respect an author that you are reading, but you may not really be connecting with them. On the other hand, if I say, "The sky is blue," you might agree with that without having any emotional component to your opinion.

Conversely, you can have an emotional response that doesn't come from a conscious thought. Imagine you're looking at a flower. You could have an emotional response to it that arises from your subconscious. For example, you could be thinking: *Oh my gosh, that flower is so pretty!*

In this case, you aren't looking at the flower, trying to figure something out using your conscious mind. You aren't trying to recall what species of flower it is, for example. You are having a purely emotional reaction to the beauty of the flower.

Physical

Most people are aware of the physical realm of health, to some degree.

Physical elements include:

- Physical habits
- Exercise
- Diet
- Well-being
- People who share your space
- Your relationships, good and bad

People usually have at least a fairly good understanding of—if not a handle on—the physical, but often lack an understanding of some of the other three elements of health. In addition, their understanding of the relationship between the four elements may be incomplete. I often see this in my chiropractic practice.

The four components of health are part of all your actions. They are involved in all the events of your life.

Picture this scene:

You are driving down the road, and you drop your phone, so you reach down to grab it. Then you look up and, all of a sudden, you see a red light—*oh, shoot*—and you know on a conscious level that you're not going to able to hit the brakes before you get to that light. Off to your right, you see a car coming at you, and you can tell it will be coming through the intersection at the same time as you. You know—on a cognitive level, on a **mental** level—you know that you are going to collide. There are going to be very **physical** consequences of that collision. Your body will be moved in a certain direction, organs may be displaced, and some injuries may occur. You will certainly experience **emotions**— including the sheer emotion of fear. Lastly, based on your **spirituality**, you might pray for angels to protect you—or something of the like.

You can see that all four components are a part of this situation, as well as every circumstance of your life. Your state of health will be determined by the health of these four elements.

What Is Your State of Health?

Where are you at spiritually, mentally, emotionally, and physically?

As we've already discussed, it is always important to know where you are beginning. The idea isn't that you must be in a certain place to begin—on top of the mountain or deep in the valley—you just need to know where you are, in order to begin to change.

If you are on top of a mountain, then it is important to know that, hey—there are higher mountaintops, and you don't even have to go into the valley to get to them. There is always something higher. You can always raise your level.

For the person starting in a valley, the only way to go is up. Then, when you reach a pinnacle, there are more pinnacles to achieve. Know that you can raise that achievement to an even greater level. You can blow your life out of the water. You can blow yourself out of the water with what you can create.

Setting Intentions: Where Do You Want to Be?

Once you have inventoried your state of health, it is time to set your intentions. In life, our intentions can make all the difference.

For example, what is your intention for reading this book?

If you are reading with the intention of identifying with the content and actively helping your life grow, you will be much more likely to get positive results.

Read over the questions below and answer them:

- Where are you, right now?
- What are your perceived achievements?
- Where are you spiritually, mentally, emotionally, and physically?
- Where do you want to be in each of these areas?

Remember, wherever you are is okay. Don't focus on what you see as your failings; focus on your intentions. If you are in a state of depression or anxiety, then obviously, you will need some work in the mental and emotional areas of health.

Physically, you may be overweight or underweight. You may want to go outside more to experience more sunshine. You may want more exercise. Perhaps you would like to start putting foods in your body that can keep you going through the day, instead of only keeping you going until your next break at work.

Are you being empowered spiritually, mentally, emotionally, and physically?

Are you being fed properly in each area?

This is not a beating-up process. Don't beat yourself up. This is simply an honest account of where you are and where you want to be. Only after you make this assessment can you set intentions for change. Setting these intentions is crucial to the process of growth.

Look at this process in terms of seasons. Just as we have seasons of different kinds of weather, we also have seasons of growth. Everyone thrives differently in one season versus another, and that is fine. Celebrate the seasons of your life; they are necessary parts of growth. Some seasons may progress a little slower than other ones, but you must honor the process and keep going.

Let's stop here, and summarize what we've talked about so far.

As you begin to take inventory and plan for changes in your life, here are the four key points that you should keep in mind:

- Know where you are beginning.
- Figure out where you want to be.
- Set your intentions.
- Realize there will be different seasons of growth that will get you there.

Setting Goals That Arise From Your Intentions

Goals that you set for yourself should be specific, and they should come out of the intentions that you've already established.

Consider these questions:

- What intentions have you established for yourself?
- Where do you want to be at the end of this process?
- What is your highest good?

If your intention is to have the perfect body, then you are going to focus more on the physical side of health, and your goals will arise from there.

However, consider carefully: Is this your highest good?

Do you want to focus exclusively on just the physical element of health?

Through this process, my hope for you is that you realize how much the spiritual or emotional will affect the physical. Issues in these other areas can manifest physically and contribute to dis-ease. When we look at the word dis-ease, we can see that it actually means *a lack of ease.*

So, what is this lack of ease all about?

It will always tell you about something that is lacking in one of the four elements of health—spiritual, physical, mental, emotional—or perhaps, in a combination of them. You will have to look at the whole picture to get a realistic idea of your level of health.

Don't judge where you are at—I can't stress that enough. Be kind and openhearted with yourself.

Initially, you will set certain intentions and goals, but as you begin to move ahead, your achievements may end up surprising you. As you grow, the whole process will be affected by your growth, and along the way, you may well shift your intentions and goals.

For example, perhaps I want the perfect physical body. However, as I move forward toward this goal, I might end up seeing more about myself than I did initially: *Oh, I see that I need something else. I have more stress in my life, mentally and emotionally, than I realized. I really need some help for that from an outside source. Moreover, I see now that, when I work on these areas, my spiritual side is also going to grow.*

Instead, maybe I have a wonderful belief in a creator, maker, and father—a God—and have set intentions in this area, not giving much concern or attention to my body temple. My goals may be to help others spiritually, but as I learn and grow, I may discover more: *Oh, if I give my body more attention, I see that improving my physical health can only help me make a bigger difference in the spiritual area. I can actually better help others if my physical body is stronger and if my thought processes and my emotions are in balance.*

WORKING TOWARD YOUR HIGHEST GOOD

In my life, some of my best teachers, along with some of my hardest lessons, have come to me in some of the hardest times in life. I went through many years of depression and anxiety, feeling small, and so much less than I knew in my heart I was meant to be.

Life is full of times of loss. Loss can be experienced in relationships, in a broken heart. Loss can be due to the death of a friend or a family member. The situation that you are experiencing right now may involve loss, and if so, you know for yourself how strongly it can affect your physical, mental, emotional, and spiritual balance, and your well-being. You may be wondering why you are experiencing this terrible loss.

We think of life as *happening* to us. However, in reality, life is not happening to you—it is happening around you, and you are participating in it. You choose to participate in this thing called life, and you choose how.

You should ask yourself:

- What is my level of participation?
- Am I a silent wallflower-observer?
- Am I actively engaging?
- Am I a leader?
- Am I a follower?

Don't think of these words as labels; they are just questions to check what's going on inside you. If you don't like what you find, now you have the wonderful option—because we are all given free will—to change. We have a choice. You have the choice to change if something is not to your liking.

Everyone is given blueprints to build on from childhood—we'll talk about these more in the next section—and some blueprints are not structurally sound. They may be poor frameworks to build on and need to be changed. For example, some of us have frameworks that have arisen from the opinions of friends and family members telling us what we can and can't do in our lives. When you hear these voices, remember that you have a conscious choice.

What decision will you make regarding how you participate in your life?

These friends may truly be saying these words out of love. They may believe they are saving you from being hurt. Some may be trying to keep you from trying to achieve something because they are jealous, but many times, a friend just doesn't want you to be unhappy if you fall short.

How do you respond?

You can either accept what the words are saying, believing that you shouldn't try, or you can forge ahead anyway. Either way, you will be using your belief to direct how you participate in life.

Take honest inventory of yourself, your intentions, and your goals and use this inventory to make your choices about how to participate in your life. From that place, you can make an informed decision.

It's time to take your inventory, and ask yourself: *What do I want to do with this information?*

For instance, I was told—and it was ridiculous—by my peers that I was never going to grow up to be anything. Somehow, it got stuck subconsciously in my mind. I had adopted that belief, and I was living my life according to this paradigm, although I was largely unaware of it.

Even after I had achieved certain things in life, I still felt: *I'm never going to grow up to be anything*—even though I had already grown up to be something.

Once I was consciously aware that I was still operating off this negative paradigm, I did something about it. I made it like coal for a locomotive. I answered every *you can't* in my head with *I can!* Every negative thought I had was like coal for my fire, for my locomotive. That locomotive grew strong and fast. I hope my story helps to encourage you to do the same with the negative voices in your head.

Always remember that you have a choice. You decide how you participate in your life.

Perception: A Definition

It is funny to me that throughout my life—I'm talking from age seven on—I've been asked, "What's the meaning of life?" Adults and children have asked me this question, in one form or another, more times than I can count.

Even at age seven, I remember answering, "Your perception."

That is exactly what it is. We all have frameworks, usually given to us by our parents, which we have built our lives upon. As you've already read, I like to call these frameworks our blueprints because it is from these plans that we build our lives, the way a contractor builds a house. We are given this blueprint as children, and it incorporates everything that our parents have imprinted upon us.

I quite often hear, "You are just like your mom," or "You are just like your dad."

I personally love to hear these comparisons. I love my parents; they are wonderful. However, I know that not everyone has had such wonderful experiences with their parents. Regardless of your background, if you don't like the blueprint that you were given, you don't have to build that house. You can wipe out that blueprint and create a whole new framework. Or, you can build an addition instead of wiping out the whole thing. It's your choice.

The meaning of life for you is your perception. You may begin to see what your perception is when you look closely at your blueprint.

What does your blueprint look like?

Are you working on a healthy framework with a strong foundation?

You may not be so sure that you like your blueprint enough to want to begin building a framework on this foundation. You may not be ready to build because you need to change your plans. That's fine. Go ahead, change your construction plans, and start somewhere that feels right.

A Small Part in a Bigger Plan

Why are we here?

This question is another one that comes up often in our minds, in conversations, and even in dreams.

What are we here for?

Only you can answer that question, Reader. I believe that we are all here to raise universal consciousness for the greater good.

What is your greater good?

We all have contributions to make, and it matters. Before each election, I often hear people talking about whether their vote matters. Of course it does, because it is the collective, made up of individuals, that determines the outcome of elections. A collective can do magnificent things—just look at what ants can do together.

I look at humanity as if we're all part of an ant farm. As an ant on that ant farm, you have a specific job and duty. If you don't perform your duty—I hate the word duty in this context, but it's applicable for the ant farm—if you don't perform your duty, the link is broken. Because you are not pulling your weight, someone else must do your duties as well as their own.

Ant communities are so magnificent. Ants are tiny beings, you know, but when you've got ants all working together, they create these wonderful hills. We are all just like ants in an anthill; we each have an important role in the community. If each person doesn't pull their weight, then the hill falls apart. When you do pull your weight, you are contributing to the universal consciousness.

What is your idea of the highest good—peace, love, or joy?

When you do your part, you are contributing to your idea of the highest good.

Life Is Open-Ended

For each of us, life will appear either open-ended or dead-ended. I am here to tell you, for certain, that life is open-ended.

What does this mean?

When you are really trying to work on one of those four areas of your life—physical, mental, emotional, or spiritual—and you encounter a roadblock, it may feel like a dead end, but it is not. So often, when people hit a snag as they are trying to raise the bar in their life for their highest good, they immediately call it a failure.

Remember this: *Failure only happens if you fall down and don't get up.*

When setbacks happen, you are being given an opportunity for growth. Within the experience, there is always a lesson that you can use later down the road, in a future endeavor. It is a lesson within a lesson. Not only are you getting the gifts of what you are trying to achieve, you are also getting an idea of how to smooth out the process for every achievement you have coming in your life ahead.

As Tony Robbins wrote in his 2007 book, *Unlimited Power: The New Science of Personal Achievement*: ". . . there's no such thing as failure; there are only results. You always produce a result. If it's not the one you desire, you can just change your actions, and you'll get new results."[1]

Life is open-ended, not dead-ended. It is okay to head in a direction that doesn't ultimately end up fruitful for you. It's okay if your efforts don't yield the result that you were looking for. It's okay—unless you stop trying. If you were to stop, that would be true failure; you won't go anywhere further.

If you understand that life is open-ended, you'll keep moving. You can move in a different direction if you need to.

Do you feel afraid?

If fear is keeping you from moving, remember that there are only two degrees between excitement and fear. They are similar vibrations. If you are feeling fearful, then change two degrees off to the right or left, until you find excitement.

Remember: *There is no such thing as failure; there are only results.* Never stay down; always get up. Keep walking. Weather the storm. There is another season coming.

OUT OF YOUR HEAD AND INTO YOUR HEART

One of my favorite wise sayings is: *The head without the heart is like a tyrant. It controls everything.*

---

1   Robbins, Tony. *Unlimited Power.* Simon & Schuster, 2007.

When the head is in control, there is basically no room for passion. In turn, the heart without the head is like a small child wandering around aimlessly. The heart is easily distracted by *ooh, squirrel!* moments.

The idea of unconditional love lies somewhere between the head and the heart. Both are needed. You must realize where you are coming from. If you are coming from an open heart, which is a wonderful place to reside, that's amazing. But an open heart can lead sometimes to the perceived negative of enabling. Try to find the balance between these two as both are essential.

Pursue Passion and Find Purpose

This is your life. If you don't like the way it is going, then it's up to you to change it. Life itself has some wonderful tools available to you, and they may be right in front of your face. I hope that this book will be one of them.

The aim is to truly live your life, not just get through it to get to the finish line. Live it. Embrace it. Enjoy it—both the ups and the downs. Find your passion and it will lead you to a purpose-driven life.

Remember that blueprint we talked about?

Your parents, friends, support system—whoever is important in your life—they want what's best for you, first and foremost. They might want you to be a professional football player, an author, a doctor, or a lawyer. They may want you to learn their trade, perhaps to enter the family business. They want you to be a success, and they have their own definition of success.

In the beginning, the blueprint is important for us because we need to learn, and we want to learn as much as we can. We are sponges as children. As we get older, however, we start deciding which way we want our life to head.

Whenever you have a choice in front of you, if you don't make a decision, be aware *that is a decision*. At that point, your decision is to open yourself up to whatever the world wants to throw at you. I encourage you to see what you want, even if you know you can't get there right away—if you need specific training, certifications, schooling, or mentorship, for example. Hold the idea, first and foremost, and later, you will figure out how to get there.

The training part of this equation—well, that's the easy part. It is knowing where you are heading that is the hard part. Embrace the process.

Challenge some of the blueprint ideas that have been given to you, and see if they are applicable to you in your life. See if they fit the real you, not a formal version of you, or a definition that was given to you. Make conscious decisions because life is about decisions, and you are in control of them.

It can be difficult to go against what other people think is right for you. Our perception of our status in society can affect how we feel about ourselves, emotionally and mentally. However, it really doesn't matter what other people think. It truly doesn't. What matters is what you think of yourself.

Give yourself permission to find your own joy. You may be on an organic farm out in Colorado—if you are loving life, if you are living life fully in a grass hut, if you are happy, on a spiritual, mental, emotional, and physical level, then your life is joyous. How people find joy in their lives is a totally different book, but ultimately that's what we are here for: the pursuit of joy.

What is your joy in life?

Once you find that, you will have found your passion. So many people look for professional items first: money, security, or status. Find your passion first. If you want to be a yoga instructor—fantastic—if that's your purpose. If money is important to you, you'll find a way to make money in yoga. Maybe you'll create a video series, or start your own network of studios across the nation. Once you find your passion, everything else will fall into place. Your purpose will become apparent, and you'll find a way to satisfy all your other needs.

When I was sixteen years old, I talked to a millionaire. I told him that I wanted to know the secret to being rich.

He asked me, "Why do you want to be rich?

I answered, "Because I want ten houses."

Shaking his head, he replied, "You can only live in one."

My analytical brain said: *He's right. So, I don't want to be rich.*

Many years later, I revisited this conversation in a meditation. I reframed my thoughts about being rich. I thought: *Yes, I want ten houses. I will live in one, and nine deserving people can live in the others.*

If you want to be rich, if that's something that's important to you, you may have been led to believe that this is not a worthwhile goal. Money is not evil, but a lack of respect for money can be. If you respect money, then it will serve not only you, but also other wonderful people in this world. It's what you make of it.

Emotions Are Friends

We have a variety of emotions. Love is the wellspring of all positive emotions, giving rise to courage, joy, and other positive feelings. The opposing force of these positive emotions is fear. Fear leads to depression, anxiety, and the other lower-feeling emotions that weigh us down.

There's energy behind emotion that either lifts you up and empowers you or weighs on you and brings you down. It is important to become aware of these energies. Think of them as colors.

Think of a palette that a painter uses. Think of all the different colors on your palette that you can pull your brush through.

You might only use some colors once, and some you will never use, but they are all there; they are all available to you. Look at the available emotions, the array that you have, and you will see that every one of them has a power. They have a color, a hue, and a vibration to them. If you are constantly picking colors that aren't brightening your life, there is a lesson in that for you.

That lesson might be found in the company you are keeping or in the thoughts that you are thinking.

Take a moment to consider what colors you are painting with your own thoughts:

- What are you saying to yourself?

- Are you empowering your brain with the thoughts in your own head?

- What are the colors of your elevator music, the background music of your mind?

- Are they empowering, or are they weighing you down?

I was all but homeless for about a year of my life. I lived in the Virgin Islands in the woods. When you read that I was homeless, you might be thinking: *Oh, my gosh. That's the worst!*

However, this was in the Virgin Islands—a beautiful place full of palms and sunshine, waves, and fishing. It was incredible. I was a homeless person in paradise.

To that point in my life, I had never felt more alive than I felt during this time of homelessness. All the responsibilities of society were taken off my shoulders, and I was left with the simple joy of living. So, when I woke up in the morning, rather than worry about where I needed to go, how I was going to get there, or who I was going to be with, I'd open my eyes and just say my prayer to God or express my gratitude to God for that moment. It was amazing.

The colors I was painting with during this time were simple, peaceful, and beautiful. Such simplicity. I came to understand that life is simple; we make it complicated. If you can, find ways to de-complicate your life and paint with those lovely, positive colors.

Head or Heart

Is your approach from the heart, or from the head?

I can only speak for myself and you can only speak for yourself, Reader. I always felt that I came from my heart. I certainly have always wanted the best for myself, my family, my mom, dad, and other loved ones—and for the world as well. This has always been in my heart.

I've always felt that my approach was from the heart. But I'm laughing to myself now, because as I write these words, I realize that, for most of my life, I was deep in my head. I was so deep in my head that I couldn't really appreciate the simplicity of the heart. My heart had to experience the world for itself.

I was always looking at my life in terms of failures, under-achievements, or unfinished business. You need to recognize when you fall short of a goal, to be sure, but if you get it in your head to focus only on those things, you will derail.

Derailment is exactly the right word for what happens next. It's just what it sounds like. You are heading down the train track of your life, smoothly, and suddenly—*boom*—you get hit and now, you are off the track. Well, the solution is simple; you just need to get back on track. First, however, you need to *know* that you are off track.

When you derail, if you stay in your head, then you will stay derailed. You must get back into your heart to move forward. Your heart always comes back to the same place—the source. The heart knows, ultimately, where you need to be.

We have come to the end of this first chapter. Before you move to Chapter Two, check in with yourself:

- Where are you right now?
- Where do you really want to go?
- What do you want out of life?

- How can you help yourself get what you want?
- What do you want to gain from reading this book?
- How can I help?

In closing, I share a quote by Ted Morter. About seven years ago, I attended a seminar and heard Ted Morter, Jr. speak of his father.

He quoted his father, saying: *The only difference between a rut and the grave is depth.*

CHAPTER TWO

The Power of Words

WHAT IS YOUR YOUR INTENTION?

What is your intention?

Are you aiming for a particular destination?

You may have financial or career goals—or perhaps you want to be a good parent, or have a fulfilling romantic relationship. If you don't have a clear idea of how to get to your destination, that isn't unusual. However, you do need to know where you're coming from before you can effectively move forward.

When you meet obstacles in your path, or traumatic situations in your life, don't react until you ask yourself: *Where am I coming from?*

For instance, let's say you caught your spouse being unfaithful. Think about where you might be coming from at this point.

You could be:

- Feeling anger
- Feeling insecure and fearful
- Feeling love and sadness at the same time
- Assessing how you might have contributed to this situation
- Wondering if your attention had been recently wandering from your spouse

All these feelings are totally appropriate; there is no judgment. You simply need to ascertain what your feelings are.

Where are you coming from, and what is your intention?

Your intention is either going to take you to your destination, or it's going to help you create another destination that may be even more meaningful. Pushing through this process is vital to get to the most meaningful goals.

It's like when you are working out, and you just have one more repetition. You don't think you are going to be able to lift that last weight, but you try anyway. You just push yourself through it. Invariably, you will find, in that very last push, the most benefit. The biggest rewards are found in this kind of *intentional power*.

Love or Fear?

The emotional state itself is sponsored by two main intentions—love or fear. All other emotional adjectives can be traced back to one of these. For example, courage can be traced back to love; infidelity can be traced back to fear.

You can think of it as a tree. The words are the branches of the tree. All branches come back to the trunk to form one solid face.

Which tree are you climbing?

Are you climbing the tree of love, or are you climbing the tree of fear?

Again, the words you choose to describe your emotions and intentions will tell you the answer. Fear comes from jealousy and other negative thoughts and emotions—the negative vibrations and energies.

After you assess your situation and discover where you are, it is a beautiful truth that you can choose a different path.

These two trees are quite different, but it is possible to move from one to the other. You can change your direction. Say you find yourself climbing up the tree of fear and you don't like it. You know that you don't want to act from a place of fear. Once you discover this, all you need to do is switch your intention.

How do you do this?

Well, let's take the example of infidelity once again.

If someone you truly love has been unfaithful to you, you will begin with: *I really love this person, and I feel so hurt.*

You can choose to come at this situation from anger, which is a branch on the tree of fear, or you can come from understanding—on the tree of love. Wherever you have begun, you can switch.

You can get the results that you want by coming from a healing perspective. You must realize that healing can never take place when you operate from a position of fear; it can only happen through love. That is really what I want to get across here.

We all want to heal. We don't want to fan the fires of fear. It is only through healing that we can grow.

Contributing to Universal Consciousness

You must assess your feelings and intentions in order to progress, but it is important not to judge yourself harshly. Some people beat themselves up daily—minute by minute— but it doesn't really help a whole lot. Harsh judgments often cause people to stall completely.

If you are thinking about your life, and you see that you are heading up the tree of fear, you might be thinking: *Oh my gosh, I really am afraid. I don't like that about myself at all.*

A lot of people will shut down right there, feeling overwhelmed. When people get overwhelmed, they tend to come to a standstill. That's when growth halts.

Think of yourself as someone that you love, a best friend. Often, we can be kinder with friends than with ourselves.

With a best friend, you listen and you don't judge. You observe them, and you offer some tidbits on how to help, but only when asked. Try to look at yourself in this way. Love with detachment. When you can come at it from this direction, you can truly come to the vision of yourself with love, but also with objectivity.

You can find the clarity and strength to say: *I don't like the intention I am setting. I don't like the direction I am heading. What can I do to change this?*

When you truly come from that place of nonjudgment, you are less likely to stay stuck in a holding pattern, walking around in circles. You can begin actually moving forward.

At that point, you are ready for some bigger questions, like: *What are we all really here for?*

We can start to understand that we are all here to help one another. When we help one another, the vibration changes. The energies grow lighter; the air becomes cleaner.

When you ask people what they would wish for, many will say: *Peace on Earth.*

It always sounds like an impossible goal, but in reality, peace is simply consciousness elevation, and the only way to do that is by one soul at a time by helping each other. In helping one person at a time, we collectively raise consciousness, and bit by bit, we build peace.

Follow Your Moral Compass

The concept of a moral compass is interesting because morality has a number of different definitions. It has a negative or positive connotation for some, and no connotation for others.

Again, check in and assess yourself. You must examine your own framework without judgment, coming from that place of open eyes and open heart.

Here are some questions to consider in your assessment:

- What is your moral framework, and where does it come from?
- How were you set up as a spirit?
- How were you raised by your parents: given love, or not given love?
- How do you demonstrate love?

Love can be an integral part of one's moral compass, and people will demonstrate it differently. Some might have great difficulty showing love; others might give freely. It isn't always predictable. If a person felt unloved as a child, they may actually over-love in their adulthood. If they were given too much focus and attention as a kid, then they might under-love as an adult as they are accustomed to being the center of everything.

A strong moral compass helps set your direction. In addition, following your moral compass helps keep you moving so you will be less likely to come to a standstill.

Sometimes you just need to start moving. In these cases, it can be best not to sit in judgment of your direction because you can always change that. That's the beautiful thing about it. You may not quite trust yourself, but you can still take a stride forward. You may not be sure where you want to go, but you can follow your instincts and move on. You may not have all the tools or support to keep going in the direction you've set, but you can trust that you will find the way, even if it isn't a straight line.

Wrong or right, sometimes it doesn't matter—just keep moving. In those times, it is especially important to have something outside of yourself for support. God is my source of support. Our wonderful teachers and mentors can keep us moving in the right direction if we are open to their help. Remind yourself that you are not alone in this process.

The only thing we are alone with is our decisions. Once you make the decisions, all kinds of help will be available from the universe, to help you move in the direction you've chosen. This process requires self-awareness.

How self-aware are you?

Consider these questions:

- Are you making decisions based on your true feelings and intentions?
- Are you just going through life with no plan, with no attention to details?

- Are you taking the time to smell the roses?
- Are you not even aware that you have choices?
- Are you listening to people who have your best interests at heart?
  Consider the source.

If you are overwhelmed by these questions, know that you don't need to understand the entire process; you just need to begin. There are many places to begin, and there is no right or wrong place to start. What I have realized is that it doesn't matter which direction you are heading in, as long as you are moving.

Many people, including me, become paralyzed when they feel overwhelmed. It keeps them from doing anything at all. Then, when nothing gets accomplished, they get frustrated and bogged down in negative thinking.

If you don't have a mentor or a direction, find someone, whether through a book like this one, through social media, or through other networking. Find someone who is positive and is already in the flow in the direction that you are heading. Get in the flow; get in the stream. Start moving. Moving is the most important part of the process, right now.

WORDS HAVE POWER

Words have the power to move your life forward, keep you in a holding pattern, or move you backwards. Your words are a barometer that will give you valuable insight into what's going on in your life. Studying the language you use can be a fantastic place to begin the process of self-assessment.

Start with considering this question: What words do you use most often in everyday conversation?

We use an incredible variety of words and their meanings are often not as clear as we think they are.

Let's keep it simple to start, beginning with *yes* and *no*.

Yes and No

Imagine being asked, "Hey, would you like to go to the beach today?"

If you answer, "Yes, I would," then your intentions are clear.

However, if you answer, "Eh, maybe," what does this really mean?

Maybe really means *no* because you are not saying *yes*. Maybe you are trying to be nice and polite.

You say *maybe,* but you are really thinking: *I have considered what you said, but I really don't want to go. But I don't want to tell you right now that I don't want to go.*

Let's look at some more words.

Should, Could, and Would

Imagine using the word *should* to describe an action or intention. If you are saying you *should* be doing it, then that implies that you probably are not doing it.

However, if you should be doing it, you should *already* be doing it. Do you see what I mean?

If it is a *should*, it is a *must*. It is something that you need to do.

Why would you wait on that?

Now, compare *I should* with *I'd like to* and *I could*.

They each have a different intention, but, if we restrict the meaning of these words to either a *yes* or *no,* they are all *nos.*

Analyze the words you are using and become crystal clear with your meaning. You will feel the difference. You don't have to take my word for it. Try it in your own life, and see how it feels, energetically. You may find more negatives than you would like, and that's okay. Don't judge yourself for those; just be clear, and this will keep you from wasting energy.

Clarity is the key here.

Let's go back to the beach question. Imagine you said, "Maybe."

The person will ask again, and this time, imagine you answer, "Not yet."

They will likely ask you once again in a little while. These exchanges involve a transfer of energy. The person is sending you love and a desire for you to share an experience with them. Your energy will eventually be reflecting some annoyance because you don't really want to go to the beach, and it is stressful to keep on hedging. This kind of interaction propagates negative energy and misunderstanding.

Let's assume that both people in this story are trying to head in the direction of their moral compass. Each time you've spoken, however, you haven't been using words that represent this heading.

If you had, you would have said, "No, I don't want to go to the beach today."

Identify the words you are using in your life, and look at what they really mean. See if you can keep it simple. Simplify your life. Life is simple; we make it complicated.

Depression and Internal Dialogues

What words do you use when you talk to yourself?

Your choices can tell you a great deal about what's going on inside you. When I was in my early twenties, I went through a long period of depression, but I had no idea that this was the case. It took me a long time to realize what was happening.

What was the reason for this delay?

It never occurred to me that I could be depressed.

I am a truly happy guy. I would describe myself as an optimistic fellow. In general, I don't think negatively. I felt bad, but I wasn't thinking sad thoughts. It didn't seem like depression to me.

In the early 1990s, I had what felt like the flu. It was like a powerful wave that would come in and knock me off my feet. When it didn't go away, I went to every medical doctor I could. I had an EKG and blood tests, including a glucose tolerance test to check for diabetes. I went to a neurologist and had brainwave and CT scans.

Of course, every test came up negative. Finally, I was at my wits' end.

What was going on with me?

My physical body was exhausted. I could barely get out of bed. Sometimes I actually couldn't get out of bed. Then if I could get up, my mind wasn't clear enough to know which two shoes matched. I was so cognitively imbalanced that I just wanted to go back to bed. I had little appetite and would sleep for fourteen hours a day. It was terrible. The only thing that would get me out of bed was work. I went through this for about three years, with some improvement in the summertime.

Finally, one day, I was sitting watching TV, and a commercial for a pharmaceutical drug came on.

These words appeared on the screen: *Do you suffer from lack of appetite?*

I remember they were in big bold letters.

I said to myself: *Yeah.*

The commercial continued: *Do you suffer from lack of energy?*

Yeah.

Are you sleeping all the time?

Yeah.

The commercial went on to name a long list of symptoms that were all mine. I sat up straighter, and paid closer attention, but then the diagnosis at the end of the commercial appeared in big bold letters: *DEPRESSION*.

I sighed: *Oh. Nope, that's not me. I am not depressed. I am not sad.*

The truth was that I *was* actually going through depression. I wasn't sad; I was working from a depressed nervous system. It wasn't until after I identified the culprit that I could start to address my problems. Again, you must figure out where you are starting from before you can set your heading in any particular direction.

All those years, I had been going around and around in circles and getting nowhere. I had been growing frustrated. I was anxious. I was becoming more panicky, and I was becoming more depressed.

When you have a prolonged problem that you can't solve, I have learned that it is common to experience these feelings. I am sure that some readers out there are feeling this way right now, even as they are reading this.

Are you one of them?

I am here to tell you that there is a solution to your problem. There is a solution to every problem.

Here is the incredible truth: Every problem is really a challenge that is calling you to be a higher version of what you are now. To follow this path, you must learn to master the language of this kind of learning.

When you can do this, you will be able to answer these questions:

- What is being shown to me now?
- What am I trying to learn?
- What am I being called to learn?

First, however, you must learn how to tune in to your own internal dialogue. Close your eyes and tune in to the language that is going through your head. It is almost like elevator music, constantly playing in the back of your mind.

In my case, I was saying some of the most horrible things to myself:

- *You are no good, worthless.*
- *You are never going to get there.*
- *Why are you even trying?*

This internal dialogue was incredibly negative and defeating.

How in the world could my nervous system, my body, my brain, and my soul respond positively to dialogue that was so damaging and negative?

What is your internal dialogue like?

Assess yourself, and listen—without judgment—to the words you are saying to yourself. Notice how you talk to yourself. If don't like what you are hearing, it is time to change the language.

Frameworks and Foundations

Where does this internal dialogue come from?

It may be helpful to understand the origin of our internal language. You need to go back to the beginning to answer this question.

When we were kids, some of us grew up with one parent or two; some had other adults in a parenting role. We also had other mentors in those early years. Think back to your childhood and identify them.

What did you learn from each person who was an important mentor in your life?

Your internal foundation was constructed in these early years, and it was impacted strongly by the people closest to you, your mentors. Parents are key, but a mentor can also be an aunt or a grandparent, a family friend, a teacher, a minister, or a best friend.

Do you have a strong foundation?

What kind of house are you building on it?

Are you building your house on sand or on stone?

Our foundations are the basis of our initial beliefs as children. As we grow, we are introduced to different ideas. We either accept them or reject them based on the influence of these beliefs.

In our early lives, we are not thinking about the positives or negatives of our positions. As young people, we are usually either rebelling against the rules or we are following the rules. We are either acting out or we are trying to please. We are governed by fear or by love.

Does that sound familiar?

Notice that, once again, we return to the idea of choosing to act from fear or love. We will return to these same ideas again and again. The big picture is beautifully intertwined and connected, and you will be able to see it more clearly as you grow.

I had wonderful parents—I still have wonderful parents—who have been amazingly supportive. Most parents want the best for their children, even if it's not an ideal parent-child situation. Parents want the highest good for their child. The way they go about parenting can be very different, but at the core, they all want their kid to be healthy, happy, and whole.

Whatever framework we are given by our parents, whether it is from fear or from love, eventually we all grow up. Then, we take responsibility for the parts of the framework that we choose to keep.

We are in control of our choices. In reality, that is all we are in control of. We are not in control of how we were brought up. We are not in control of what we were taught, or how we were taught, or if we were taught at all—but we are in control of our choices.

So, what do you choose?

Here are some questions to consider:

- Where do you get your knowledge?
- Where do you seek your worth?

- Are you choosing to interact with positive people or negative people?
- Are you hanging around with the people that you admire and want to be like?

When you are on your own journey, you don't have to reinvent the wheel to find answers to your questions. Read and interact with other people. You will learn a great deal by watching. You can hear and understand new ideas by paying attention to dialogue. You can investigate how other people have gotten to where they are, especially if that's where you want to be.

You don't have to reinvent the wheel, but you might tweak it a little bit. You can build a better fire. Keep your mind open to possibilities and seek new information. If you are not getting what you need from a strategy, don't be afraid to change strategies.

Steam Locomotives and Manure

When you are trying something new, other people may not always be supportive.

Do you know what a steam locomotive is?

In the old days, trains had steam engines that were powered by coal. Workers had to shovel coal onto the fire to heat the water in the engine. The steam would power the locomotive down the track.

Early in my life, I developed a locomotive analogy to combat negativity from other people. When anyone tells me I can't do something, I visualize it as a shovelful of coal. I hear the thump of that coal as it is thrown into the fire of my locomotive.

I think to myself: *I am going to take that coal, and I am going to throw it on the fire. I am going to use it to power my steam engine. I am moving forward.*

You can do the same.

Don't judge other people for their opinion. Often, people—especially parents—are not trying to hold you down. They simply want to protect you. They don't want you to run around in traffic. They worry about you in the big, wild world. They are afraid that you are not ready to spread your wings and fly.

When we are young, we depend on our parents to protect us, and we should be grateful that they do. When you enter into adulthood, you must make your own decisions. You must create your own flight pattern as you jump out of the nest.

You may jump out of the nest and fly. You may jump out of the nest and fall. Either way, make the decision and follow it through.

Sometimes life throws you some difficult challenges. They can come in the form of criticism from other people, as we've just discussed, but they can also come from circumstances beyond your control. I think of these challenges as manure.

It doesn't always smell good, but manure can be useful, can't it?

When I get a lot of it, I say, "You know what? I am going to take the manure and I am going to grow flowers."

UNKIND AND MISALIGNED WORDS

How well do your words express what you feel and support your intentions?

If you are currently using words that are out of alignment, you may have to change your perception or beliefs around certain words.

Stop for a moment and consider these questions:

- What words are you hearing?
- What words are you speaking?
- Are your words making you feel happy inside?

Think about when you had your first dose of love. We often call it puppy love. When you first feel love for another, you feel it with all your heart, and it is true and pure.

I'll tell you my story of first love. I was infatuated with this girl in fifth grade. It was my first puppy love, and I was smitten.

Around Christmas time, I got her this stuffed dog and this really cool perfume, which I put into a small vial and attached to a puppy dog chain. I wrapped it up and added a bow and a nice card. One day, I set the package on the desk she would be sitting in during the next period, and I left. I felt so good, picturing how happy she would be when she came in for class and saw it.

At lunchtime, I went to sit with the group that I always sat with, and there was the box on the table for me. It had horrible words written on it—like *creep* and *stalker*—and it absolutely crushed me. I was totally coming from this place of love, and obviously, this other person was not.

Words that come from love are kind and supportive. Words that come from fear knock down or destroy.

I was coming from the place of love. The person that was on the receiving end was coming from fear, and what came out of her was hate language. Now, I am not saying she actually needed to love me; a person's language can come from love without them being in love. She could have told me she was flattered, but she wasn't interested. She could have recognized that I was a good person and wished me well.

We were kids, and she probably didn't know any better, but even as adults, people often don't fully appreciate or understand the power of choice.

In any situation, you can choose to come from love.

In my puppy-love story, if that girl's response had come from love, it would have changed everything for me—at that time, as well as for my future. For me, this one experience forged a conscious belief system in me. I didn't even realize, until I got older, that this belief system had affected all my relationships.

I believed that if I fell in love with someone, that person would bash me eventually. They would say mean things that would cause me pain. They would hurt me. I believed that I could not allow myself to be vulnerable because I needed to protect my heart.

All relationships that followed were rooted in that first painful experience. I was afraid to be vulnerable because I believed it was a weakness. Now I can say, with all certainty, that vulnerability is a strength. Vulnerability begets strength.

Imagine you are building a castle, and you notice vulnerable places—chinks in the armor, so to speak. You know that someone could attack you if they got through those openings. You don't ignore your vulnerabilities.

You make your castle stronger—you build up fortitude—so that they can't storm the castle, right?

After building inner fortitude, if anyone did get through chinks in your castle, what would they find?

They would find only strength underneath.

Emotions and Perceptions: Changing Your Language

Many different emotions exist between fear and love. Some of them seem very similar but are actually very different.

For example, consider *anxiety* and *excitement*. They are very close in feeling, but they are actually very different.

So, what's the difference?

Anxiety is on the tree of fear, and excitement is on the tree of love.

It's how you color it; it's your perception. Your perception is based on your belief system and your wording. It is your perception that will take it one direction versus the other. Sometimes you need to change your language or your thinking—or both.

Once you know where you want to be, you may have to flip your belief system a couple of degrees in order to head in the proper direction.

During that puppy-love incident, I was feeling all this love in my heart. I expressed that love, and then ultimately, it was pushed in my face. It was all the more difficult because it wasn't done behind closed doors; it was in the cafeteria. It happened where all my friends were sitting. It happened where her friends were sitting. I was the laughing stock of the whole of fifth grade at that point.

In my adolescent mind, I was alternating between feeling hurt, and thinking: *Well, she doesn't know what she's missing.*

Interestingly, there was one cool benefit to the situation. At that point in my life, I was trying to find myself—as we do throughout life. I remember it was a time when everyone was getting spike haircuts. I decided to get one myself. Ultimately, I changed a great deal of my whole outward appearance, and remarkably, I became *cool*. I became one of the most popular people in school.

I decided to move from that place of pain, from that experience into a different, more positive place. This was a conscious decision.

I said to myself: *I am not going to feel like that again. It's horrible and I am better than that.* I made purposeful changes in my life.

At the same time, however—as we've already discussed—subconsciously, I was saying: *I am never going to fall in love because it's too painful.*

Think about the language of your life. You may be choosing words consciously, the way I did in this situation, and they may direct your actions. However, you may not even be able to hear the language of your subconscious, although it may well be controlling your decisions and behavior.

Context is everything. Words take on the meaning that is determined by your perceptions. A word can have a spiritual context, or mental, emotional, or physical one—or some combination of all these.

Words are powerful. They have the power to motivate, to move you forward, or detract. They can keep you in a holding pattern. They can overwhelm you and ultimately, they can set you down, crush you, and destroy you.

Words That Label and Judge

Do you use or hear words that label and judge?

There is no opportunity for growth in words like these. For example, imagine that someone tells you, "You are ugly."

You have a choice:

- You can choose to agree: *Wow, I really am ugly.*
- You can choose to disagree: *No, that's not real at all.*
- You can be kind of indecisive: *Well, I don't really think I am ugly, but I am not good looking either, so it kind of leaves me in a bit of limbo here.*

We can discuss this in terms of open-ended versus closed-ended questions.

An open-ended question would be something that would allow a conversation to continue, to perpetuate, in a variety of directions. A closed-ended question can only be answered with a single word. A closed statement, in the same way, allows for no discussion. They have finality. For people, they can become statements of identity that are difficult to overcome.

If I was to say, "I am ugly," and just attach to the idea, then I *am* ugly. We are emotional beings, and that's just the way it is, whether I am or not. If I feel ugly, then that is what I am.

However, instead of just believing that statement, I can choose to combat it. I can make a different choice.

For instance, I can say one of the following:

- "No, I'm not ugly—I'm actually good looking."
- "I'm not ugly, but there is room for improvement."
- "I am not as beautiful on the outside as I feel inside, but I'd like to change that."

When you use different language, you can adopt a different position. From there, you can take action. In my case, it was as simple as a haircut, set of clothes, and different friends. If you look in the mirror and see something less than beautiful, it's up to you to find what makes you feel beautiful.

Reflecting Your Intentions

Look at the life you have created, based on the framework you have chosen:

- Is it authentic?
- Are you living the life you want?
- Are you in a place in which you don't feel comfortable?
- Are you surrounding yourself with people who are drinking all the time, or smoking, or doing drugs?
- Do your surroundings reflect your intentions?

If you are authentically attached to your surroundings, that's fine. It is your decision—no judgment. Everything serves your highest good. If you do not like your surroundings, it is up to you to change them—and you can. It is up to you.

Have a discussion with yourself. Choose open-ended questions, and examine any statements of identity that you notice. Focus on forward movement. Focus on growth.

You are not interested in standing still. That's why you are reading this book. You are not interested in stalemates, standing still, or running around in circles. That's what close-ended questions or opinions of yourself are going to get you. Instead, keep your mind and heart open-ended.

Minds are like parachutes; they only function when they are open. Hearts are the same way, so keep that in mind. Head forward with open-ended questions. If you have been standing still, find out why. If you are going forward too fast, take some time to smell the roses and receive the wonderful, beautiful lessons and gifts that are coming to you.

Challenge and Expand Your Framework

As I said before, we have all been shaped by our parents, our mentors, friends, grandparents, aunts, and uncles. You are shaped by whomever you have looked up to during your life. Based on that framework, you were given a blueprint. When you were a kid, you began to build a house based on the blueprint.

Let's continue with this metaphor.

It is possible that this particular house is perfect for you, but it may not be. Maybe you built a mansion, and this mansion isn't serving your personal goals. You could be single and may travel a great deal, so you don't need a mansion, and it takes too much time to care for.

Maybe you built a small house, but now you have a huge family, and it doesn't meet your needs. How is your family going to fit into such tight quarters?

When the framework you grew up with doesn't suit your life, you can change it. You should change it. You can expand your house. You can improve your blueprint. You can add an addition; you can make it two-story. You can move into the yard and create an oasis.

The point I am trying to make is this: you are totally in control of your blueprint. You can make any changes that you want to make. You may have had a rough beginning, as I did, but you don't have to stay there. You can wipe out the whole blueprint and draw up a whole new one based on what you want in your life.

Making these changes can be difficult. You may start with very clear intentions. You may be excited by the prospect of building a whole new house, but soon an anxious feeling creeps in.

You may start hearing new ideas like: *Well, who do you think you are? You can't do that.*

We are talking again about the subconscious. This is fear talking. Somewhere along the way, you may have picked up a belief system that tells you: *I can't.* You can combat the language, in the way we talked about earlier.

You can alter your belief system to say: *I don't want to be in fear; I want to switch over to love.*

Figure out what love language you can adopt to help you change this belief system.

It could start very simply, like this: *Okay. I might not have the tools yet. But I know that I can find them.*

Be honest with yourself when you are assessing, but remember to check in with yourself without judgment.

You Are Never Alone

If you are putting yourself out there, creating new forward movement, and changing your belief system, you need to know that you are never in this alone. You have the support of God, or the universe—or whatever your outside source of support is—to help you move in that direction.

You are never in it alone. Ever.

What is *your* source of support?

Religion can be a wonderful tool—if you look at it in the right way. I was raised in a Missouri Lutheran church that I love very much. It gave me valuable tools for my life. Christianity is one type of religion. It is my type, and it works for me, but it may not be what works for you. That's fine.

There are many subdivisions of Christianity, and every church has its own character. I could go to ten Lutheran churches, and even if each pastor was preaching and teaching on the same Bible verse, each message might be different.

Although they are different, each message could be helpful in some way. Each pastor could be giving a different perspective, which could be beneficial. Those ten different messages, sponsored by the same reading, could all help enhance my belief system and could help me move forward.

Your spiritual source of support might not be an organized religion at all. An infinite number of options are available to you.

CHAPTER THREE

Living a Balanced and Joyful Life

ENERGY, GRAVITY, AIR, AND COMMON GROUND

There are certain truths that are simply the truth—not our perception of the truth, or our version of the truth.

In my practice, I do energy work with patients. The kind of energy work that I do deals with sympathetic and parasympathetic nervous systems. These systems both interact with the brain center, which directs both conscious and subconscious thought. We are using consciousness right now. We are sharing beliefs that are in our heads; we are aware of our opinions and how we feel.

The real magic, however, is in the subconscious.

Within the subconscious is the stuff you can't hear. This is where your belief systems are stored. It is the language of the part of the brain called the *cerebellum*. The cerebellum handles balance and equilibrium in the body.

When we are talking about subconscious thought, we are essentially talking about belief systems. There are many belief systems, and they often impact my work.

For instance, it is fascinating to me that, among the people who have come to me for treatment, some have said something like, "You know what, I don't know why I am here. I don't really believe in energy."

I always kind of laugh and say, "Well, if you lick your finger, and put it in that socket, something's going to happen, right? That's energy. It doesn't require that you believe in it because you are going to be affected by it, one way or another."

There are certain truths that are laws. They don't depend on people believing in them.

A person can say with certainty, "Oh, I don't believe in that, therefore it isn't true," and it won't change the law.

Another example is the law of gravity. If I have ten things and throw them into the middle of the room, every single one of them is going to fall on the ground because gravity is a law. It is truth regardless of my perception. An awareness of these laws can help bring power and clarity to life but, more importantly, it gives us ownership of our own power.

Are you really doing everything you can do?

If you're not aware of the inescapable truth of these laws and their use, are you really working toward your highest good?

Meeting People

In my line of work, people come to me for help. Obviously, I want to help them the best I can.

My question for each one becomes: *How can I best help this person?*

To begin, I must open a dialogue with each person. The language that we use will invariably reflect our belief systems, as we've already discussed.

I am a Christian. It is an integral part of my belief system. It is how I've been raised, and for me, it is a foundation; it is my rock. However, I know it is important not to alienate people by forcing a belief system onto them.

You must meet people where they are. There are certain truths that we all can agree upon, and this provides us with a starting point for further conversation. We need a starting point so that we can begin to move through to where we need to go, to arrive at the destination. We must all move from where we are right now.

After all, it is from this place that a person asks for help. You begin from where you are. When you're trying to help someone, you must meet them at their starting place in order to have a chance of helping them.

Back to our example: if someone comes into the office and says, "I don't believe in energy work. I don't believe in God,"

I certainly don't want to shut down my conversation with them.

We could talk about what we believe. We might discuss what is true according to each of our different belief systems. We need to come to some sort of meeting place in order to get anywhere. Talking about the truths that are laws—like energy, gravity, and air—can be just such a meeting place.

For example, I might say, "You don't have to believe in air, but you are breathing it anyway; it is keeping you animated and alive."

Or, "Whether or not we believe in gravity won't stop it from keeping us here on the Earth."

Then, we can find a meeting place from which discussion can begin.

Transfer of Energy

We are all made of energy. Again, this doesn't require a belief system. However you look at it—no matter what framework you have grown up with—this is a universal truth.

You can see it as cosmic or magic, or you can simply call it a universal force of law, like the air we breathe, like the gravity that is holding us on this earth. The sun comes out every day, whether it's hidden by clouds or not. The sun is there whether you can see it or not.

There is a law of physics called *conservation of energy*. It states that energy cannot be created or destroyed; it is simply transferred from one form to another. If you can wrap your head around that idea, there is a lot of power in it. It has an impact on all aspects of life.

Are you a pessimistic or an optimistic person? Is your glass half empty or half full?

I used to believe that a person is either one or the other. I believed that we were all born with that quality. What I have seen in life has shown me a different truth. It's pretty darn amazing. A person can start off with a glass that is half-full and turn it into a glass that is half-empty—and vice versa. This is a true example of the concept that *energy is not created or destroyed, only transferred.*

What are you putting your energy into?

What is the state of your *glass*—half-empty or half-full?

Remember, it's all about the words you use, so what language would you use to describe your energy?

- "Wow, this life sucks. It's me against the world."
- "It's me in this world, along with everyone else."
- "Life is good, and I am grateful for my place in the world."

The distinction between these is huge. Your state of energy will motivate or demotivate all your life actions.

I Am Not the Center of the Universe

Consider these basic human questions:

Why are we here?

What's the whole purpose to this?

We come upon these questions at critical times in our lives, prompted by circumstances like disease, death, or loss of a loved one. We are each led to these questions by ourselves, and I think that everyone answers them for themselves.

I can only use my own experience to try to connect with others. I try not to rock their belief systems but to share my own and come into common ground to find a good starting point.

One issue that comes up often is the existence of outside forces in our lives. For me, this is never in question. I am certain that forces greater than me—like a Creator, God, or other forces of the universe—have an active impact on my life. Something outside each of us is steering us toward our highest good.

When we are considering the basic human questions posed at the beginning of this section, the existence of an outside force will deeply affect our answers.

If there is no Creator and it is just me, then what am I here for?

If I am everything and everything is me, then what is the meaning of my life?

If I am everything, then there is no need for anything. Ultimately, my contention is that, without outside forces, there would be no need for human experience; we would just be living and dying, and that would be that.

We all need something outside of ourselves, a point of light outside of ourselves, to compare ourselves to as we grow. During the night, we need to know that day exists. If nothing tells us what light is, we could forever exist in darkness without ever realizing it.

As human beings, we search for deeper meaning, and I believe that is because we inherently know that there *is* a deeper meaning. It is instilled within each and every one of us. It's in our DNA.

Then the question becomes: *What is this deeper meaning?*

We have created all kinds of constructs and belief systems within our societies—God, Buddha, the Big Bang. No matter what your beliefs are, we are all part of one world; there is a commonality between all of us. Personally, I think there is magic in all of it.

I think it is the similarities, rather than the differences, that we should focus on. We spend too much time trying to disprove one another's belief systems. We have many more similarities than differences. Again, we need to start from common ground.

As you've read, I've been through some tough times. A large part of my life was spent going in and out of depression. I'm a thinker and a super analytical person. I often over-analyze. While I was in that depressive state, I was deep in my brain, deep in my own mind, in my own belief system. I was so deep in my own reality that I didn't have room for anything else. I didn't allow anything else to come in at that time.

I had created my own world, and I was the center of my universe.

Let's go back to words and language again. When I stepped away and started thinking about it, I listened to what I had been telling myself all this time. It was like being in a closed room, surrounded by elevator music that I had created—and much of it wasn't very nice. I discovered that I didn't like what I had been saying to myself. I didn't like what I was hearing.

So, at that point, I had a choice:

- Did I want to listen to this elevator music that I knew inherently was wrong?
- Did I want to continue using a voice that I didn't like?
- Should I continue playing a record that didn't truly represent me?

I knew I needed to change records. When I did, my belief system was strengthened, and I was put on my path.

One day, I was going through a period of super depression. I was in my early twenties and couldn't get it together. My world was spinning. I could barely get out of bed. I was deep in my head once again. I managed to get outside, just to get sunlight and breathe some fresh air.

Then something inside of me said: *Get out of your head.*

As I did, I found myself staring at the ground. Then, I realized that I was staring directly at an anthill. Gradually, I noticed that there were ants coming out of that hill and that there were ants coming to that hill. There was a whole amazing system there, right in front of me. I hadn't really paid attention to things like that since I was a tiny little kid.

This new awareness was such a striking experience for me because it was right under my foot, literally. It was all right under my nose, so to speak. Then as that realization came to me, I started wondering what else I had been missing. I closed my eyes, and I started hearing birds that I hadn't noticed before. I started to feel more like part of the world, rather than feeling separate and insulated. I started to feel like it was me *with* the world, not me *against* the world.

WE ARE NOT ALONE

You are not alone. You are not the only one on a journey in this world.

If you were actually the only one, there wouldn't be much to figure out, would there?

The game would kind of be over, wouldn't it?

You would be by yourself, the only one that mattered, and that would be it. You would be done. All questions answered.

If you look around, however, it's not just you. Life is complicated, and there are many things that we don't understand—many, many things. It would probably take several lifetimes to be able to understand it.

So, if I am not the only one, what does that mean?

Let's go back to the anthill. In that moment, I became aware of the multitude of processes happening all around us—the birds, the ants, animals and other life, the forces, chemicals, atoms, and molecules—so many things around us that we don't sit around deliberating or pondering on the average day. We are not consciously aware of most of them, but they are still going on around us.

If you are stuck in your head, you will be especially unaware.

Let yourself feel the world around you. It's not us against the world. We are part of the world. At my most isolated, it felt like the weight of the world was coming down on me. I felt like I always needed to press against the world. I didn't understand that it was my own weight, my own thoughts pressing down on me.

The world is not against me; I am an inseparable part of the world. It's me *in* the world, not the world against me. Although we can see some of what's around us, there is much that we can't. Not everything is as it seems.

Creator, Orchestrator, or Grand Designer

The more we realize that we are alike as a species, as a human race, the more it helps us get to the bottom of what we are looking for in life as individuals.

Too many people spend their time looking at the differences between ourselves—our religions and our cultures, foods, dress, skin color. It's ridiculous. If you take all of that away, everyone has a heart, and everyone has the same organs. Essentially, we are much more similar than we are different. It's fine to remember the differences, but focusing on our similarities is what is going to help us get to the bigger questions of life.

Let's talk about the existence of a Creator. We can call it a grand designer, an orchestrator, an architect, God, Allah, or Buddha. I do believe in the existence of a Creator. I am not trying to step on anyone's sensibilities, but let's find a place we can create unity on this subject.

What if we could take all these possible names, for the sake of argument, and simply say that there is a Source?

Set aside whether it is Buddha or Allah, as well as the details of any framework of belief. This Source would simply be a beginning and an end, something outside of ourselves. If we can all agree on that much as a species, then the semantics won't matter. If we can just get back to the Source of it all, we can find a place to come together. We can focus on the idea that we are simply here together for a purpose. Love one another, whatever your belief systems are.

When I was in chiropractic school, we had a cadaver lab. I had a good friend in my class who was an atheist and didn't believe in much of anything.

If you cut open any cadaver, it looks the same inside, whether it was a male or a female, black or white. The same organs are there, blood flowed to the same places, and the brain looks the same. The organizational intricacies of the body are the same in every single cadaver. The lungs are here, the liver and spleen are there, and the heart is in the same place every time.

My friend was amazed. He marveled at the organization.

He said, "You cannot deny it; there is a grand orchestrator. There is a masterful hand in all this."

Consequently, by the end of the program, he was not an atheist anymore. Sometimes, religion can actually bring people together, rather than separating them.

Wonderful Guides

There is so much information nowadays, making it is easy to experience information overload. Computers, phones, audio, video, and media of all kinds are all around us. We have so much stimuli, and it can be overwhelming. In addition, the wealth of information makes it seem like it should be simple to find the answers you seek, but it isn't always that easy.

We often need help from other sources.

Guides and teachers are all around us, if we only know where to look. As we have discussed before, nature can sometimes be an easy and effective way to open your mind. You can step outside and watch what is going on. You may see birds nesting. You may see critters gathering food. You may hear the sharp warning chirps birds make for their protection, guarding their flocks.

There are guides all around us—God, best friends, peers, teachers, children—if we can only tap into them. Even your worst enemy can be a guide. Anyone who cares enough to offer you an opinion can help guide you toward answers.

Why?

When someone has an opinion, it can cause you to make a choice that you were hesitating to make.

You may be on the fence about an issue, or you may have been avoiding making a response to a matter. Whenever someone else expresses an opinion or asks a question, their words can force you to move directionally in some way, changing from one point to another.

Remember that energy isn't created or destroyed; it is only transferred?

Whenever you move directionally, you are transferring energy. You might be using the energy for movement; you might be making a different choice or taking a new stand. Some of my best mentors, my best guides, have been people whose way of thinking is completely opposite mine.

An antagonistic opinion can help you see a different perspective. Not only can this help you to see another's point of view, it can also help you to more fully articulate your own position. Even when you strongly disagree with someone, having a respectful discussion can help both people understand each other and themselves, as well as the issues, better.

There are many guides who are available to you in the written form—books, articles, and blogs, for example. Again, if you use them in a constructive way, as we've described, that's fantastic. Keep your mind open. You may sometimes feel as if you've heard it all, but there are always new sources of information.

Life experiences, however, are the most valuable sources by far.

Travel. Go to different areas to view different cultures, meet different people, and figure out what makes them tick. Talk to people and listen to new ideas. See what matches with your belief systems. See what goes against them. The thing about belief systems is they are always changing—like energy—and there is always a way to improve. You are always moving toward your highest good.

As a Christian, I do believe in angels and demons. I believe that they represent a broader spectrum of balance. You can call it *yin* and *yang*, or light and darkness. From the experiences I have had in the world, and from what I was taught, this balance exists.

Meditation is a powerful tool. For me, meditation and prayer are synonymous. They both take you outside of yourself to find balance. They help you find a place where you can feel that you are an integral part of the world—not you against the world.

Find something outside yourself to connect with. If you are only looking to yourself, and focusing exclusively on what you can taste, feel, touch—good luck! You will only get a small part of the story.

The Universal Law of Balance

Once you connect to the various elements that can function as guides for you, you will need to create a balance between your being and theirs. You will need to find a middle ground, a fulcrum, to foster understanding and create balance. We are not in this alone.

I am forty-three at the time of the writing of this book, but I can remember my childhood days on the playground. I remember loving the teeter-totters. Some people call them seesaws. I remember I would go out there by myself, and I would sit on one of the teeter-totters and wait for someone else to sit on the other end so we could play.

Without someone else, it's hard to play on a teeter-totter, making it a fantastic analogy for balance. At this young age, the teeter-totter shows us how we need balance, and we need another person to help experience balance.

When another kid comes out on the playground and gets on the teeter-totter, we go up and down. Everyone is having fun. Each person always wants to be on the high end of the teeter-totter. When you are on the high end, the other person is down on the ground, and they push off hard so they can get back to the high point. While you are playing, you are helping each other stay balanced. Eventually, however, you know what will happen. Inevitably, one of the parties will lose interest and step off. The other person will come crashing down.

Sometimes, isn't life very much like that?

It brings to mind a question of trust.

Think about the relationships you have in your life right now, and consider these questions:

- Do you trust the person on the other end of your teeter-totter?

- Are they going to jump off, or are they going to stay and help you balance?

- You have friends, family, lovers, perhaps a husband or wife, and kids—are they sticking with you on the teeter-totter? Are you sticking with them?

- Can you balance your own needs, your selfishness, enough to enjoy the ride?

- Are you just going to jump off, and leave the other person hanging?

The moral fiber of the people involved will help shape the answer to these questions. In the teeter-totter analogy, your belief systems can provide that fulcrum. Belief systems help us determine for ourselves—not based on anyone else—the best way to balance ourselves.

Which side are we on—the high part of the teeter-totter, or the low part?

It is all about finding that fulcrum. It becomes essential for balance throughout our lives. Balance is harmony. Balance is peace.

There are so many different names for balance, and there are many facets of balance. There is emotion attached to every word that we could use to describe balance, and they are all valid and true. I believe balance is the essence of life, the answer for how to get in and out of this life alive.

Find your balance, wherever that is, in all areas of your life. Find it within yourself, in your relationships, with your outside sources, and in all the other areas of your life. A few examples are given in the sections below.

Balance within Yourself

Is your biggest battle the battle within yourself?

I'm not good enough—I am good enough—I'm too good: Can you see the teeter-totter analogy here?

We always need to seek balance.

Balance in Your Financial Situation

Financially, do you have too little or too much?

The balance may have to do with how you manage issues associated with money. Survival, satisfying basic needs, generosity of spirit, and appreciation for what you have— these are some of the issues related to finances that could impact your balance.

Balance in Relationships

What kind of balance do you have in your relationships?

- Are you giving as much as you are getting, or are you taking all the time?

- Are you pulling from people, from their energy, from them, draining them?

- Are you enhancing their lives as much as they are enhancing yours?

- Are you a grateful receiver?

It's all about finding that balance.

Balancing Your Relationship with Outside Sources

Consider your outside sources—for me, this is God—are you giving as much as you are given?

Life is a precious gift; are you living it to its highest potential?

If you are not, then you must get right on it and get back to balance.

Find out what that balance is for you. It might take a little while, and that's okay because life is a journey.

What do you do once you find balance?

Life would be boring if that was the end of the story, but it isn't. Just like the teeter-totter, balance must be continually maintained. A little up, a little down, up and down. This is the way of life.

In a relationship, people often use the term fifty-fifty to describe the balance between them, implying that each person must be giving and taking equally all the time. On the teeter-totter, in this situation, you can picture each person perfectly balanced on a level horizontal board.

This rarely happens, right?

In a real relationship, one person might be having a great week, and they might be able to pull the load of two in the family that week. The other person might not have as much to give that week. The next week, it might be reversed. Over time, if people are doing their best, there is a kind of balance created.

Life is like this. Balance is an ongoing pursuit.

THE HUMAN EXPERIENCE AND THE GIFTS OF LIFE

This human experience is very much an emotional experience.

Everyone knows emotions. We each have a full spectrum of emotions, from good to bad. One moment, you could be excited and happy in a new relationship or a new job. In another moment of your life, you could be having heartaches in a relationship and may have a job that isn't at all fulfilling.

The human experience is designed to enjoy every single piece of it.

It might seem like we are meant to seek only the good and to keep seeking until we have the ultimate, which some would describe as *peace on Earth*.

What if we had it? What would that look like?

Holding hands, happy, and singing?

Okay, what do we do after that?

Life would essentially be over at that point. What else would we have to do?

We need the peaks and the valleys. You can't differentiate the common ground until you've had the extremes. You can't understand happiness without sadness. You can't understand joy without pain. It comes back to the yin and the yang law of balance. We need both yin and yang to appreciate where we are.

In the heart of whatever experience you are going through, ask the questions that reflect your own participation instead of focusing on what's been done to you.

How are you participating?

How are you showing up in your own life?

When I was in the deepest part of my depression, wondering what it was all about, an answer came to me in one word: *patience*. I didn't fully hear it right away, and even after I heard it, I didn't know how to find patience.

How do you teach someone patience?

One way to do it is to give them a bunch of hardships. It's not the only way, but it is one way. Experiencing hardship gives you a way to practice patience.

Enjoy the Moment

Take time to smell the roses whether life is difficult or not, whether you feel great or bad. Take the time to truly experience the emotional state that you are in. Try to remember to ask yourself about the manner in which your emotions are coming to you, and how they make you feel.

Do you notice recurring themes?

Are there lessons that you are learning?

With modern information technology, everything moves faster than ever before. In this fast-paced world, we must remember that we are not meant to hustle along without thought or feeling. We are not little *Ants Marching*, like in the 1993 Dave Matthews song.

Taking time to smell the roses is a colorful cliché, but it is accurate. If you are not taking time to enjoy life, then you are minimizing the joy of it. You are not savoring it.

Instead of roses, think about a piece of chocolate cake.

There are different ways you can eat the cake:

- You can wolf it down without thinking about it.
- You can eat it one bite at a time using a fork.
- You can use your hands and stuff the whole thing in your mouth.
- You can eat slowly, noticing the different flavors that hit your mouth.
- You can eat it but be thinking about the calories—feeling bad with each bite.

Maybe you are on a diet, and you've told yourself: *I can only have one cookie today; that's my allotment.*

However, you don't need to eat the whole thing in one gulp. You can take it bit by bit, enjoying every single bite. Look at all the events of your life in this way.

During the birth of your child, you can think: *Oh, this is messy—gosh, I've got to raise this kid. I'll have bills for healthcare, formula, diapers, education, and so much more, and my spouse can't work if they stay home with the baby.*

Alternately, you can think: *Gosh, I just brought this beautiful thing into the world!*

You can experience the feel of the new baby's skin and scent. You can celebrate the baby's first poo, and think about all the joys that are going to come—teaching them to speak and sing and how to ride a bike.

It is your choice because life is a choice. It is based on how you want to look at it.

Is this a burden, or is this a blessing?

Opportunities for Growth

There is a poem by Jane Eggleston that includes this verse:

> *Thank you for valleys, Lord,*
> *For this one thing I know*
> *The mountaintops are glorious,*
> *But it's in the valleys I grow.*

I have thought about this idea throughout my life. Although I appreciate the beautiful words, I believe that it is not only in the valleys that we grow; it's on the mountaintops too. I am not going against what the author is trying to convey, but as with anything we read, it's our perception of words that matters.

My perception is: *OK, if it's in the valleys I grow, maybe there are other lessons to learn elsewhere.*

After all, if I am growing here in the valley, then what am I doing at the opposite places?

What if I reach the top of the mountain, and I see a higher mountain to go to, do I have to go back to a valley to learn?

In my perception, there is always some place higher to go. A valley could be seen simply as a lesser mountaintop. This perception, rather than looking down, keeps me looking up for the next higher adventure, the next greatest good.

When we are trying to understand something, we often look at an issue as black or white. While I appreciate the value of both sides, I really enjoy the gray. Gray areas occur where the two sides mix, and there is magic in both of them. For me, the gray areas bring me closer to the fulcrum of the teeter-totter. A gray area can give us more if it gives us the best of both worlds or teaches us a lesson from both.

I want to learn as many lessons as I can. I want to be the best person I can be. I strive to be the most effective I can be in this life.

At the end of this life, I want to be able to say, "Wow, that was a fulfilling life."

Enjoy Every Bite

When I was about twenty-one, I was working for a surf shop in Virginia Beach. When business was slow toward the evening, we would look at surf magazines, and we'd read about all these pro surfers who travel around the world to beautiful places. We'd look at pictures of beautiful people, exotic foods, and incredible waves, and we would all sit around and daydream together, saying to each other, "Oh my gosh, how great it would be to do this."

One day, something clicked inside me, and I said, "You know what? Why can't we do this? Why can't I do it? Maybe I am not good enough to be a pro surfer—I am not—but I love surfing. What's keeping me from traveling and seeing all these beautiful places?"

I made a decision right then. I was going. I had no idea where I was going, absolutely no idea, but I made a very firm decision. The universe responded, and I felt the shift. God, my angels, and all my support people came in to support me.

I gave a month's notice. About a week later, a friend, whom I hadn't seen in years, came into the shop. She was super-tan and her hair was sun-streaked. When I asked her where she'd been, she said she'd been in St. John, in the Virgin Islands, for two years.

I knew in my heart, right there and then, that's where I was going. I didn't have a detailed plan and didn't know how long I would stay, but that was okay. I was making a forward movement, breaking free of the paradigm of just sitting around, thinking how great it would be to go places.

It was an incredible experience. Initially, I didn't have a place to stay, and I wondered, for a long moment, what I was going to do. I was presented with an opportunity to freak out or be okay.

It was a choice:

- Was I going to sit there and freak out?
- Was I going to swallow the cake in one sitting without tasting it?
- Was I going to breathe in the fragrant air and figure out what to do?

Then it occurred to me: *I'm in paradise.*

There were options; there always are. I decided I could sleep in the woods. It was awesome. There were some challenges with that, but there were also amazing joys like learning how to live off the land, learning the fruits that were edible, and learning about natural remedies that could be found in the woods.

Living like that broke life down into its simplest form. It took away money, societal standards, and class systems. We were all as one. It took me back to the heart of what's important. Survival was a focus in the beginning, and once survival was taken care of, it was all about the meaning of life—and enjoying life.

At that point, I had the means to sit in the woods and enjoy each sunrise and sunset. I had a place to live. I enjoyed good health. I could enjoy having the energy and ability to look around at sea shells. I could look out at bays and go snorkeling and surfing.

Life changed. I was enjoying each bite of that cake.

How are you spending your life?

I would say a lot of people are frozen in place. They are not moving anywhere because they are indecisive. They feel overwhelmed because they are afraid of making a wrong move; therefore, they don't make any move at all. I have been guilty of this myself. That is what depression is, really; it freezes you in one point in time and keeps you there.

Reader, if you find that you are in one of those states and you are stuck, I encourage you to move. It doesn't matter which direction you move.

You will figure out whether it is right or wrong, because life is going to show you—your spirit will guide you, or your Source will show you. The beautiful thing is that you can always make a new choice if you need to.

Lack of movement is more dangerous than moving in a *wrong* direction.

Sometimes we become overwhelmed after monumental events in life, and it causes us to freeze. It can be heartache; it can be joy. It is always important to do a quick little mental wrap-up so that we don't miss any of the gifts that were given to us during an overwhelming event, whether it is perceived as good or bad.

There are always gifts. What doesn't kill us makes us stronger. Glean everything that you can from the experience. Don't miss anything. Don't minimize the importance of your gifts.

Maximize everything. Get all the marrow. Participate in all the soul reflection you can. Be honest with yourself.

Pause and check in with yourself when you have an important life experience, but don't allow yourself to freeze for long. Life is waiting for you to move forward and keep on learning.

CHAPTER FOUR

We Are Only in Control
of Our Choices

YOU ARE NOT THE CONDUCTOR: LEARN TO SEE YOURSELF AS PART OF LIFE

You are not in control of life. This fact can be hard to accept.

You are a part of life. You are in the mix. On the train of life, you are not the conductor.

This goes back to something we talked about in previous chapters as well. We are *in* life. Life doesn't happen to you; life happens around you. It is your choice to engage at any particular moment in time.

For instance, you could be sitting on the subway or the bus, hearing a conversation. Maybe it's someone on the phone, or maybe two people are conversing. They might be talking heatedly about something, and they could sound frustrated or sad. Listening, you may have some sort of emotional attachment to the situation.

You have a choice at that point:

You could offer help. You might say, "Oh my gosh, I've been in that very situation and this is how I handled it—maybe that will help you."

You could just sit back and listen. You could reaffirm for yourself, thinking: *Wow, I remember what that felt like, and I can see how I moved through that and I can see that I learned from that.*

Life happens around you, not really to you. You are like a chess piece. You can choose whether you want to engage at any point or you can sit back and relax, observe, learn, and grow.

You are not in control. As we discussed previously, we all need something outside ourselves—God, Buddha, the universe—for perspective and sometimes, to lean on. Very little about life is in your control, maybe 3 percent. If it's not in your control, you must learn to let it go. This is why you need something outside of yourself. We can't do it by ourselves.

Gazelles and the Lion

Ever since I was a young boy, I have always been captivated by the African jungle and the savannah of the Serengeti. I always found lions especially fascinating.

Once, when I was working at a hotel, I had a conversation with a man who was a CEO and general manager. This was a man I greatly admired. I had noticed how confidently he carried himself and was intrigued by the person he had become.

I asked him, "How did you get to where you are?"

He told me that he had come from humble beginnings, just like me. He talked about the characteristics of gazelles and lions in Africa. He thought of the world as a lion and we people as gazelles. In the savannah, if you are the slowest gazelle, obviously, you are eaten. That lion is going to catch you.

In my mind, that slow gazelle is the equivalent of the person who is lazy, the person who just sits there expecting life to come to them. The fast gazelle is the person who goes out and takes life by the horns, so to speak. The fast gazelle is on the ball and makes good decisions and choices. The fast gazelles are motivated.

The fastest gazelles are running ahead of the pack. They are not only running away from the lions, but from the rest of the pack of gazelles as well. There is danger in this because if you get too far ahead of the pack, you won't know what's going on; you won't be learning. You will only see ahead of you and won't have full awareness of your friends or of your surroundings.

In other words: *The pack is where it's at.*

So where do you want to be?

You want to be right in the middle because the lions will pick off the gazelles on the outside. If you are in the middle, you can be safe as well as engaged in life. You don't have to be the fastest or the slowest gazelle. In the middle of the pack, you can learn and you can grow while being protected.

Rowboat or Yacht?

If you have determined that you are not where you want to be, you are ready to head out into your own future. It is an exciting time. Now is the time to prepare for your journey.

Imagine you are planning a trip. You will have to answer some basic questions.

First, how do you get there?

- Walk
- Drive a car
- Fly
- Paddle a canoe
- Take a rowboat
- Sail a yacht

Second, you know that you can't make this decision until you know where you're headed. Obviously, if you are going around the world, you can't drive a car, and the rowboat is probably not going to work. If you want to sail the oceans of the world, neither driving nor flying will be appropriate.

You will need other equipment besides a vessel. If you have a gas-powered boat, you will need fuel. You've got to be prepared for all kinds of conditions.

In the seas, you've got to be ready for winds that could come up out of the calm. Storms can be rough, overpowering, and scary.

In life, the equivalent of these changing conditions would be the number of unexpected challenges that come at us—like heartache, a death in the family, or a physical infirmity.

Are you prepared?

If you are in a rowboat, you will need to sink it and find yourself a different ship—perhaps a nice size sailboat. A sailboat won't need gasoline, so you don't have to worry about running out of gas and the winds will be there to help you, not hurt you.

Take a few minutes to know your intentions and direction, and start to make your plans. Here's a page for you to begin:

Write your plan

_____

_____

_____

_____

_____

_____

_____

_____

_____

_____

_____

_____

_____

_____

Control Your Choices

Many people are unhappy on this Earth because they are holding too tightly to this idea of control.

Control is an illusion. The only thing that you are in control of is how you live your life, how you conduct yourself in this life. You are in control of your choices and that's all.

You are not in control of what other people think of you or do to you. You are not in control of situations that life throws at you. You are not in control of any of these things, but you are in control of how you respond to them. You are in control of your own choices, good or bad.

For instance, if someone called you *pretty*, how would you react?

Would you believe it and accept the compliment, or would you minimize it?

If someone called you *ugly*, how would you react?

It wouldn't feel good. You might wish you could control that person and keep him from saying such things, but you can't. However, your reaction is your choice. It is your belief system that will direct your responses, so you are in control in this moment.

Your reaction reflects how you feel about yourself, inside and out. This will be key, as will the way your belief system defines *pretty* and *ugly*.

You may be able to say in your heart immediately: *I know I am not ugly.*

Alternatively, you may believe the person who called you ugly. Your belief will direct your behavior in either case.

RUNAWAY TRAINS

Try this exercise:

1. Hold up your two hands.

2. In your right hand put all the things that you worry about in life.

3. Remember what we established in the last section: You are not in control of what life deals you, of what other people think of you, of how other people behave. Now look at your right hand and ask yourself: *Am I in control of any of this?*

4. It is likely that the answer will be *no*. Most of the things we worry about are not in our control.

5. Now, look at your left hand. Place in that hand the things you do control. These are your choices. They are your responses to what happens to you. At any one moment, you are only in control of about 3 percent of life.

Our lives can feel like a series of trains moving. At times, we are walking next to the train tracks, watching the trains pass by. At other times, we are walking on the train tracks. Life throws things at us and catches us off-guard. Sometimes you can be overwhelmed by multiple events. It can feel like an emotional roller coaster—or a runaway train.

Imagine that there is a train coming directly toward you. You have a real decision to make at this point.

Here are some options:

- You can stay where you are in front of the train.
- You can put your hand out and say, "Stop."
- You can fight the train with all your might.

These options aren't going to be very effective, are they?

The train is going to run over you. You will be squashed or dragged along to wherever that train is going. Your motion is entirely out of your control. You will not stop moving until the train stops.

Let's look at this situation again. A train is coming at you, and you have no control over it. However, remember, you do have control over something—*you have control over your choices.*

There is one more option. Do you see it?

If a train is coming at me, I can step off the track. I can let the train go by, and then get back on the track. This is my choice.

I can't control the movement of the train, but I can control my choices. This is an effective analogy for life. I can't control much of what happens in my life, but I can control my actions and reactions.

In martial arts, there is a discipline called Aikido. Aikido techniques use the energy of the attacker. When an opponent moves toward you with aggression, you can sidestep and allow their body to pass by you. You can gently push them and guide them away from you, using their momentum to put distance between you and them.

You may not be able to keep someone from attacking you, but you can make choices that get you out of the way. This is the same idea.

Our Choices Define Our Lives

Life is a series of things that happen either to us or around us. As we've discussed, you choose your actions and reactions.

Life is a series of choices. You choose whether you want to get out of bed. You choose whether you want to talk to someone at the supermarket. You choose how you want to engage with the world. You might have an interview, but you can decide if you want to go to the interview or not.

Our choices will define our lives, in one way or another. If you spend all your time worrying about all the things that are out of your control, you'll be miserable throughout your life. If you have the courage to make choices that move you forward in a direction you want, your journey will take on a magic all its own.

Understanding that you have choices will keep you busy all your life.

Feeling Your Way

We are all spiritual beings having a human experience, and not just a human experience, an *Earth experience*. The Earth experience is an emotional one. It's based on emotion.

We are headed now for a philosophical conversation. If it doesn't resonate with you, that's fine—just keep reading on.

I've studied people all my life. I've watched them and admired them. They are fascinating and mysterious. During my life, I have seen a puzzling trend. I have seen people who have amassed great amounts of wealth as well as acclaim and fame, and yet they are not happy. This includes highly educated people—doctors, lawyers, and scientists.

I ask the question, "Why aren't they happy?"

It's because the Earth experience is an emotional one. There are a lot of people who are very smart, but the human experience is not in the head. It is in the heart. Although you need the intellect to process emotion, if your focus is in the head, you will miss the boat. People who focus in their heads are out of balance.

This Earth experience is an emotional one. You can't think your way through life. You can't use your intellect to process your experiences and gain a true understanding or true happiness. You may have many successes in your life, but you will miss the mark, no matter how you try.

I am a Virgo and analytical. I take everything apart. When I learned that the intellect wasn't really getting me where I wanted to be, I started to delve into the emotional side of me.

I began to ask the right question: *How does that make me feel?*

Think about your own nature, and do a little self-assessment. If we break it down into a metaphysical realm, we have *the head* and we have *the heart*.

Which one are you coming from?

The head without the heart is like a tyrant, as we've talked about before. It will tell you what you are going to do, how it is going to be. It will keep you in line. There will be no deviating from the path, and there will be no creativity.

The heart without the head, as we've discussed, is like a little kid wondering around randomly, just looking at the beauty of the world.

We must find the middle ground. The magic is in between. I believe that unconditional love lives in the point between the head and the heart. That's when balance—again, there's that beautiful word *balance*—is created.

Heartache and Regrets

Somebody once asked me, "Do you have any regrets?"

I thought hard about it, then I said, "No," and I truly meant it.

However, I'd have a different answer if you were to ask me, "Have you made any really bad decisions?"

The answer would be, "Yes, absolutely."

I've made many mistakes, and some of them have caused me pain, but I don't regret any of my experiences. I have found that heartache goes hand in hand with growth.

Life is easy and smooth when you don't take risks, when you don't open your heart.

However, that's not where growth and opportunity lie. When you're sailing smooth seas, you will still grow incrementally, but real growth happens when something totally blindsides you, like love. It happens when your heart is wide open, and you can feel that you are coming from this place deep inside you.

Sometimes, of course, these experiences end in painful crashes. We've all had our hearts smacked. We've fallen in love and felt amazing, only to have it turn out horrible. I've had my heartaches, and so has everyone else out there.

Well, the lessons that are learned from a broken heart are painful, but they are exponentially large. In fact, some of my biggest heartbreaks have resulted in some of the greatest triumphs in my life. In a way, these heartbreaks have been mentors to me because I learned so much from them.

Did it hurt like hell?

Absolutely.

Would I ever regret it?

No.

Three Percent is Plenty

Remember the two-hand illustration?

Hold up your two hands. Divide everything in your life into two categories. Place everything that you have no control over into your right hand and everything you control in your left hand.

For example, you might be worried about your finances—is this under your control?

It depends how you think about it.

If you are waiting for an inheritance check to come in the mail, or for your lottery number to come up, these things are out of your control.

However, what about getting a job?

This *is* under your control. You can go out and get a job. It might not happen right away, but you can at least search. You can apply and you can interview.

Times are tough—I get that—but excuses are rampant. When something is within your control, don't make excuses. Make choices instead. You can only focus yourself if you are truly committed to this process. Once you focus on your intentions, you must put your actions behind them.

One more financial factor to consider: Are you living outside your means?

Many people spend more than they have, using credit cards and incurring other debt. If you are one of these people, that is something within your control. You can start limiting your debt right now.

Be honest with yourself. See where your choices are negatively impacting your life and make changes.

Your Illusions

Someone who spends more than they earn is living an illusion, in a way. They may get used to spending as if they make a much larger salary than they bring in. Often, people are not what they appear on the outside.

When I was an undergraduate in college, I lived in a bad part of town. The college was beautiful, but everything surrounding it was pretty run down. The house next door had a front porch that was misshapen—it was slanted at nearly a forty-five-degree angle—and the rest of the house was in shambles. Every morning, a guy would come out of that house, unshaven, wearing these funny, green slippers. He'd be holding a big cigar in one hand and a forty-ounce bottle of liquor in the other.

Each morning, he would sit on that ramshackle front porch, wearing his funny, green slippers, smoking his cigar, coughing constantly, and drinking his forty ounces of alcohol. When he was finished, he would go back inside his house.

When he went out, you would have had trouble recognizing him. He looked dapper. He was clean and close-shaven, in a three-piece suit. Anyone who saw him after he left that broken-down house would think he had it all together.

It's a great story and very true. A lot of us create an illusion for the outside world. Some of us even fool ourselves.

There are many different illusions. It is an illusion to spend more than you earn. It is an illusion to think that everyone else has it easy. It is an illusion to believe that life is against you.

Everyone is going through the same thing. Remember, we are part of life; life is not against us. Life is not punishing you; the universe is not punitive.

Are there any illusions you are maintaining?

Are you trying to keep up with the Joneses? Is that important to you?

It is not important to the universe.

It takes energy to keep up an illusion—precious energy that you could be using elsewhere. Stop expending energy just to serve illusions.

BROKEN HEARTS: PAIN, JOY, AND GROWTH

Who hasn't had a broken heart?

I think just about everyone out there, on some level, has had their heart broken, either romantically or by a friend, a sibling, or a parent.

There is an instinctive reaction to heartache. What you probably do—subconsciously—is to clutch your heart because you want to protect it, and you hold it securely. It is natural. When something hurts and we want to protect it, we grab it and pull it close. Of course, the heart is behind the chest wall, and you can't actually grab it. However, this is an appropriate metaphor for what we tend to do emotionally.

Imagine you are clutching your heart tightly.

What would happen?

You would not be allowing the heart to function the way it should; you would be stifling it. Whatever is coming into the heart would have nowhere to go. You would be effectively hardening your heart. You think you are protecting it, but putting a fortress around your heart only keeps it from working properly.

From an anatomical standpoint, you have different chambers within your heart. Keep in mind that the heart is three-dimensional and so is everything around it. Clutching the heart energetically will compress it. If you visualize this, you can see that squeezing the heart would keep it from pumping.

Let's consider your heart as your emotional center and explore the metaphor further.

What would happen if you compressed that emotional center, the way you tend to clutch your chest during times of heartache?

You would only be limiting your heart's emotional potential.

There is a better way. Instead of reacting to heartache by clutching your heart, let the heart air out. Imagine a situation in which you meet someone, and they are not as wonderful as they originally appeared to be. You can simply allow the heartache to pass through the heart. It will still be painful, but you can allow it to pass through.

If you let the feelings pass through, you can glean the good from the bad without hardening your heart and limiting its potential.

Don't build a fortress. It only limits the next love opportunity that comes your way.

Remember, control is an illusion, and this applies to the heart. You can't prevent yourself from getting hurt. Sometimes people put a great deal of energy into avoiding feelings, thinking that this puts them in control of heartache. This is an illusion. You must allow the heart to feel pain as well as joy because there are lessons in both.

If you really want to protect your heart, then set it free. Allow it to be out there in the open. This is where it is truly protected because it is where it is meant to be. It is the nature of the heart to be open, to feel. The nature of the heart isn't just to feel only the joy; no, it has many chambers. It processes the pain as well as the joy. That is the grander lesson in the bigger picture. We want that lesson. We want it because we want to grow.

That's what life is all about, right?

It's about taking all the spices of life, and this is one of them. If you do allow your heart out there, without clutching it to you, you will feel pain, but the pain won't last as long. It will allow you to move to the next lesson, toward your next joy.

The heart is a powerful tool. A lot of people give the brain all the credit—and it deserves some credit—but the heart deserves at least an equal amount.

Note that I've referred to love and heartache here, but it doesn't have to be a romantic situation. It could be another kind of heartache, another kind of pain. Anger, for instance, is a common feeling, and it always results in pain. No matter what kind of pain you are feeling, allow your heart to feel it. Then, let it go.

Listening for Resonance

I think life is an absolute miracle. It's a miracle with so many different facets. You never know where your next lesson is coming from. You also don't know who your next teacher is going to be.

Don't discount children. You can get some of the greatest life lessons from a child—from a two-year-old, from a four-year-old. As anybody who has children knows, kids are no-nonsense. When they say things, they shoot straight from the hip. They don't have filters, so some of the things they say can hurt.

Some people only look to gurus. They wait for an answer from a lofty source and can easily miss a kid calling them on their cell phone with something profound to say.

The point is don't limit yourself. You never know where wisdom is coming from. Don't miss the lessons. If you hear something that resonates, look at it and hold on to it.

When I was a kid, my mom used to recite this proverb:

> *Two natures beat beneath my chest.*
> *One is cursed; the other is blessed.*
> *One I love; one I hate.*
> *The one I feed will dominate.*
>
> ~Author Unknown

This goes back to the yin and yang, again.

Which part are you feeding?

Are you focused more on one side?

Are you allowing either one to come in?

You never know where your next lesson is coming from.

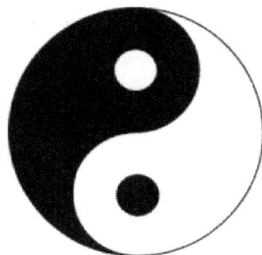

Yin and yang are important in the Chinese culture. Visually, yin and yang are represented as a circle with a white side and a black side. In Chinese medicine, it is about balance. You can't have the good without having the bad.

A lot of people want peace on earth, but what would that really look like?

Think about the yin and yang symbol. Peace on earth would be all white, and there is no balance. Now, I am not saying peace on earth wouldn't be a great thing—of course, it would—but both sides would have to be working together to create that peace. You've got to have an opposing force to know what you are fighting for, so you know why you are creating the balance.

We need both the yin and the yang, the good and the bad, the light and the dark. Evil versus good—pain versus joy—there are so many ways to look at it.

Who Are Your Mentors?

If you are trying to make a million dollars, is your mentor someone who has a million dollars?

Have they done it for themselves?

If you want joy in a relationship, are you talking to a mentor who has been divorced five times?

Shouldn't you choose someone who is in a happy, healthy relationship?

It's not about judging someone because they have been divorced five times. They might truly have it together and may have learned important lessons. The point is that it is important to choose mentors wisely.

Select people who are living the way you would like to be living. A good mentor isn't just someone who has a PhD or other great acronym behind their name. It's someone who sees and experiences the world in a balanced way. In my opinion, that's what makes a fantastic mentor.

Beginnings Do Not Determine Our Course

We all have a beginning, and we all have an end. Where that end is, I have no idea, but we can trace the beginning back to our birth and our upbringing. Whatever that experience has been for you, you have been imprinted by it. It has left a mark.

However, you have a choice. You choose whether to follow that imprint. For instance, you may have started with virtually no resources. You may have had no money and barely enough food or clothing. You still have a choice. You can change the circumstances of your life.

I have met some people who have come from the hardest, harshest, most humble beginnings and are now some of the most powerful, enlightened, and joyful people I've ever known.

Conversely, I have met people who have come from the best upbringing conceivable. They have all the money in the world, they have had every opportunity, and they have loving people all around them. Yet, some of these people are unhappy and out of balance. Some are addicts who are in AA, or who have been through rehab more than once.

Our beginnings don't determine the course of our lives. No one is being punished by being dealt a lesser hand. You still have all the opportunity in the world. You are just as responsible for your outcome as someone who has been dealt a better hand. We all have equal responsibility for our lives.

Keep the train on track. There is always a lesson to learn. Don't judge a book by the cover. There is light and dark in every single one of us, and sometimes, if you have the courage to see the light when it is very dark, you can make the light brighter.

CHAPTER FIVE

Happiness Is a Choice

HAPPINESS: INTENTION, VISION, AND GROWTH

What is happiness, and how do you achieve it?

Human beings are always trying to find out what happiness really is. It is common for people to have false belief systems concerning happiness. Let's look at the words that we use to talk about it.

Here are a few examples:

- *People are either generally happy or generally sad, and you can't change that.*
- *Some people are just born happy.*
- *People are happy if they are raised in a good family.*
- *If you have enough money, you will be happy.*

I've had friends who have come from humble beginnings, and they are some of the most integrated, wonderful people I've ever met. They are truly happy. Conversely, I have friends who have had love and all resources available to them, and yet they constantly rebel and complain. They are some of the unhappiest people I've ever met in my life.

The truth is: Happiness is a choice.

Happiness is a choice that you make. It is about your intention, your vision, and your growth. It is not dependent on where you are from; it's dependent on where you are going.

Ego out of Balance

Let's face it, we all have an ego. It is not a bad thing; it is a good thing. The problem comes back to the universal law of balance. When the ego gets out of balance, the path of your life can easily get off-track, and your mission can be compromised.

How does the ego get out of balance?

It happens whenever a person starts to feel that they are the center of the universe. If you feel this way, you'll be able to see it in the language that you use in your mind. You need to notice the way that you talk to yourself. Your inner dialogue will tell you a great deal.

For example, I am a chiropractor. My mission in life is to help people heal in mind, body, soul, and spirit. If my ego were out of balance, I might start using this kind of language: *I am the only one who can do this for people.*

Of course, this is not true. It greatly exaggerates my importance and puts the focus on my ego, when we are all here to help one another. We are all here to do our part.

Check in with yourself.

- What is your ego telling you right now as you are reading this?
- Is your ego out of balance?
- What does your inner dialogue tell you? Is it making sense, or are you creating an illusion?

Don't worry if you find that your ego is badly out of balance. Many times, if you just take the time to notice your ego is out of balance, you can easily fix it. This is all a part of the process of growing as a human being.

Just as we need *bad* to understand *good,* just as we need darkness to understand light, we need to understand the unbalanced ego in order to understand how to have a balanced ego. Balancing the ego is an integral part of our happiness process. Make the choice to maintain a balanced ego.

Co-Create Your Happiness

Although I have said that happiness is a choice, in truth, we are co-creators in all aspects of our lives. You are a co-creator of your happiness, and you are always working with a higher force.

As I have said before, I am a Christian. My higher force is God. Yours may be different. No matter what it is, your higher force is a point of reference that will help you in every facet of your life.

In the Bible, everything begins in the book of Genesis. In it, God had a desire, a genuine need. He had a choice to make, and He chose to be a creator. Then it is said that God toiled for seven days. He created the night, the day, the sun, the moon—the universe. Later on, the Bible says, we were created in God's image. Because of this, we were all instilled with the desires that God has, as much we can understand them here in this human experience.

In my personal interpretation of this, we were born as equal creators. God created this wonderful playground—the heavens and the earth, the sky, the animals, and the birds. Everything here is beautiful.

Next, it became our job to find happiness within this beautiful universe, by co-creating. A lot of people just leave it to the systems that are already in place to determine their happiness.

Have you heard people say that every religion tries to put God in a box?

In fact, systems try to put God in a box with definitions, rules, and narratives. In these systems, followers often depend upon this box for their happiness.

Here is my realization: *There is no box!*

God *is* the box! God is what is inside the box, and God is what's all around the box. So really there's no box except the ones we create. My thinking includes happiness as a choice we co-create, *outside the box.*

These systems have value. I am proud of my background as a Christian, and it adds to my perception, but I have come to understand that you should use your life experiences to make it real for you. If it doesn't resonate in your heart and soul, it won't do you a lot of good. Remember that life must be understood by the heart, not the head.

You must continue to check in to see: *How do I feel about that?*

Co-creation doesn't require your belief system. You are doing it whether you believe or not. You are a co-creator. If you are not seeing the happiness that you so desperately want and deserve, then you can create it.

The Washing Machine

I often think in terms of analogies, as you may have noticed.

This analogy came to me one day in a funny way. I was in a real hurry, as we all are from time to time, and I didn't have clean clothes for work. I threw a load of laundry into the machine.

When I am busy, I don't have a whole lot of patience. I was sitting there, just staring blankly off into space. I was waiting impatiently for this wash to get done so I could throw it into the dryer—otherwise, I would be late for work. That was the conversation going on in my head.

Then, there was a magic moment. I was staring at the washing machine and I realized something profound. In the machine, while the clothing is spinning, the center of the washing machine is static—*it doesn't move.* Everything else spins around it. You put clothes in and they spin around, but the center never moves.

I had a moment of clarity, and it opened new questions for me:

- Was I putting myself in the center?
- Was I expecting my dirty laundry to get clean magically while life spun around me?
- Was I standing still—with things left undone and my personal relationships uncared for?

If I was always putting myself in the center, no wonder the laundry was coming out dirty. The bigger picture became clear to me. I had to put God in the center. When I put God in the center and I stepped away, I released the burden and allowed the dirty laundry to be washed in the natural motion of the machine.

In effect, this is stepping away from my ego, saying: *I am not the center of my universe.*

When you put yourself in the center, you are putting a huge burden on your shoulders that ultimately can't be realized, and the wash will not come out clean. You must put something outside of yourself into the center of the machine. For me, it is God.

In your washing machine, what cycle are you using?

Are you on the quick or normal wash?

Okay, you may have to change your mode at certain points in your life, but you must choose wisely. For instance, when you are talking about huge life decisions—transformational decisions—these are times when you don't want to be on the quick wash. You need to enjoy the ride and make sure that you have a nice long time to process the information fully.

Patience is a virtue. It takes patience to make sure that the important wash comes out really clean.

FINDING HAPPINESS IS A TWO-PART PROCESS

So many people crave happiness but still don't receive it. In their hearts, they are begging for it and praying for it, but it never comes.

Are you one of those people?

Happiness is a two-part process, and you must complete both parts. You must ask for it, and then, you must receive it. The first part may be the most difficult for some people. It is hard for some people to ask for help. We are stubborn. We don't want to put people out. Other people in our lives already have full plates; we don't want to be a burden.

When life circumstances happen that leave you overwhelmed, you must ask for help. That is the first step.

The second step may be difficult to understand: How do you receive happiness?

Imagine that I am having a hard time with something, so I ask: *Oh, God, please help me.*

I have completed the first step. Now, I sit back and nothing happens. Help doesn't come in any way that I am expecting it to come.

What do I do now? Maybe I throw up my hands and then, start a new conversation: *Oh God, you are not listening to me! Why aren't you helping me?*

This is an example of failing to have the awareness for the second part of the process. You first ask for it, but then you have to receive it. To understand this, think about what keeps you from receiving help and happiness once you ask for it. There are many possibilities.

Here are a few of them:

- You might be impatient and aren't willing to wait for help.

- When the response you get isn't exactly what you envisioned, you might reject it.

- There are many different excuses you might have for not accepting help.

- There might be a belief system in the way.

- Deep inside, you might feel unworthy of help or happiness. If you don't feel you are worthy, you are never going to get it.

Consider how good you are at asking and receiving help. Now is a good time for self-assessment.

What Does Happiness Look Like?

Happiness is a personal thing. You may have heard that beauty is in the eye of the beholder. It's very true. Happiness is in the eye of the beholder as well.

Happiness for some might be a small log cabin in the middle of a beautiful forest with a lake full of fish and clear running water. Another person's idea of happiness is being on Wall Street as the head of a big company where they are in charge. They are running the show, making lots of money, driving nice cars, and having nice things.

There is nothing wrong with that. Everyone is different.

You must ask yourself: *What do I want?*

You can't get to your destination if you don't know what the destination is. A lot of people treat this part of life as if they're skipping a stone across the lake.

They throw the stone out on top of the water and see where it lands, thinking: *If I get two jumps, that's great. If I get five jumps, that's even better.*

When you use this kind of strategy, you are not making a decision. You need to make purposeful decisions. Happiness is a choice, but you've got to know what it looks like for you, and then decide how to get there.

The Right Direction

There are so many directions to turn in life.

How do you figure out which way to go?

Here are some questions that can help you begin to decide:

- What kind of thinker are you, right-brained or left-brained?

- Are you creative, or are you more of a nuts-and-bolts person?

- What is your passion; what makes you?

- What excites you and motivates you to get up in the morning?

- Do you like numbers; does crunching numbers make you happy?

- Do you especially enjoy helping people, being a caregiver?

Gather information about yourself and figure out what direction feels natural. After you decide where you want to go, you must start planning.

The Tools You Need

Perhaps you've decided you are most happy as a caregiver. Okay. Perhaps you are considering becoming a doctor. Obviously, that is going to take schooling, and you will need to plan. Now is the time for more questions and some research.

What kind of tools will you need to become a doctor?

Education is one tool. To become a doctor, you will need an undergraduate degree, plus medical school and further training. You may need specific certifications or licenses—these are other kinds of tools. Money, another tool, will be required.

You learn the requirements, and then, you have to meet the requirements. You must determine which tools you need to get you to your end destination—happiness. However, you must reach point B before you can jump to point C. You can't move straight from A to C. Plan your path out well.

After you have researched the requirements, look at them critically, and perform another self-assessment:

- What does your inner voice say?
- Are you built for this process?
- Are you capable, at the core?
- In the end, will it make you happy?

To you, *President of the United States* might sound like a wonderful position. Personally, I know I couldn't do it. I don't have the patience, I'm too stubborn, and I couldn't do it effectively.

You need to assess yourself.

What do you really want?

What will make you happy?

It is your choice.

When you are doing this self-assessment, don't allow money to dictate your options. Think more about your nature and consider what you require to be happy.

Consider this checklist:

- Am I smart enough for this position?
- Do I have the right work ethic?
- Am I in the proper place geographically?
- Am I in the proper place in life?
- Is the timing right?

- Do I have new responsibilities—a marriage, a child— that will make it impossible to pursue this path right now?

Once you go through your checklist, and everything looks right, it's time to put the project into real terms.

Seeking Abundance

Don't be afraid to seek abundance instead of settling for something small. Let's use a very simple example.

Let's say that I am hungry, and I say to my friend, "Hey, I'm hungry."

My friend says, "Oh, okay, no problem, I've got an apple right here."

They offer me the apple, but in my mind, I am thinking: "I said I was hungry. I need steak, I need something of substance, and this person is offering me an apple."

I say again, "I'm *hungry,*" and the person looks at me inquisitively and says, "Yes, here, here is an *apple.*"

You know that you want something more, but you haven't asked for it. You could take the apple and still be unsatisfied, or you can explain that you are ready to go for dinner.

Don't be afraid to seek abundance in your life. Think about what you really want before you make a plan to go forward and don't accept less than that.

When starting a new venture, sometimes people wonder: *Should I start small, or should I be ambitious?*

If you shoot for the stars, you will at least get to the moon. My advice is to be ambitious. If you shoot big and you hit it, that's great. The whole universe is yours. If you miss, you are still halfway there.

Raise your expectations for yourself. The beautiful thing that I have found about using this simple principle is that you are likely to surprise yourself by what you are capable of doing.

You will not only amaze your friends and your family, but more important, you will amaze yourself. Whatever you thought you could do, you may blow that thought out of the water. Then everything will proceed exponentially because the next time you try to achieve something, you'll blow that out of the water, too—and so on, and so forth.

PATIENCE AND GRATITUDE: GOOD THINGS COME TO THOSE WHO WAIT

Patience: everyone needs it, few of us truly have it, and it is a lifelong process. If you are already good at it, you can always be even better at it.

Patience is one of those qualities that pays dividends for your entire life. The better you understand it, the richer your life will be. Your relationships will be more fulfilled; you will have better friendships, better business interactions, higher self-esteem, and a more balanced ego.

Patience is just like any other skill. It takes practice.

So, how do you learn patience?

Practicing Patience

Start by being patient with yourself and with the process of learning. No one ever becomes good at something without practice.

If you have no patience, life is going to present you— constantly—with the opportunity to learn to be patient. The opportunities will show up in a number of ways: some pleasant, some very unpleasant. If you are struggling with patience, remember that there are gifts in everything, including the struggle. There are lessons in everything.

Learning to be patient will help you in all areas of your life.

So how do you learn it?

You can't learn patience quickly. You can only learn it when the finish line is not directly in front of you. Then, you can choose to enjoy your life, even in the waiting. Patience, therefore, is a choice.

Struggles in Shifting Sand: Leaps of Faith

When I was younger, I used to place permanency on just about everything. If I was in a depressed mood, I would tell myself that it would never end. I was sure that nothing was ever going to change. I was going to feel that way forever. This was just a lie.

How many things in your life, Reader, stay the same forever?

Almost nothing. The whole idea of permanency is a fallacy.

This lack of permanence is part of the beauty of life. If nothing is permanent and everything is shifting in life, we must shift and grow along with it. It is part of the nature of the struggle. It is this struggle—in all the shifting sand—that leads to growth.

It's the struggle that makes life worth living, makes us better, stronger people, in whatever areas of our lives that we are working on.

So, change the question in your mind from *What is permanent?* to *What am I learning?*

This process takes a little more patience. It requires that you step back and look at a much bigger picture. In my case, although I was feeling sad in this moment, I could now see that this moment was only one grain of sand in a huge beach. It was only a tiny fragment of my life.

I asked myself: *Is this going to matter in five years?*

Probably not. Therefore, it doesn't make sense to base my entire reality on this moment in time. Once I could take the permanency out of my perception, I could make a different decision. With this new understanding, I decided that I was going to smell the roses. I was going to take control of my choices, and move forward.

Friedrich Nietzsche wrote in his 1888 book, *Twilight of the Idols*, "That which does not kill us makes us stronger."

It is absolutely true. Have faith. Have faith in yourself, and then dare to have faith in something bigger than you. It is one of my life's missions, and I think it is at the core of our DNA, making it the mission of each of our lives on some level.

Expectation Versus Gratitude

One thing I have learned in life is that God doesn't give you any more than what you are already grateful for. However, our expectations for life often far exceed our level of gratitude. I've been guilty of this throughout my life.

I don't care if all you have in life is a blanket—it's something to be grateful for. If you are not grateful for that blanket, you are unlikely to get anything else. You are putting the cart before the horse if you place expectation before gratitude.

If you are stubborn—like me—this may be a harsh lesson. However, it's also very rewarding. When I truly grasped it and opened my heart to it, it was hugely rewarding. I realized that I had lived most of life, as many of us do, in a state of expectation.

I graduated college. I got my certification in chiropractic. I felt that I deserved—I expected—to be picked up by a good firm. Then, I expected to find the perfect building to create my own practice. After that, I expected to have lots of patients because my heart was in the right place, and I deserved it.

Wrong.

First of all, I had missed the most important part of the equation along the way, and that was gratitude.

For example, I should have been grateful that I had the ability to go to school at all. Wow, that's huge! Now, I am grateful for it. Afterwards, when I had school loans to repay, I should have been grateful that I was able to get those loans in the first place—they got me through school. When I found a paying job, instead of being disgruntled about the part of my salary that went to paying back the loans, I could have been grateful that I now had the opportunity to pay back the debt.

All along the way, I had focused on wanting and needing, instead of being grateful. I always needed more of this and more of that. I felt entitled. This idea of entitlement is widespread.

What are we actually entitled to?

We are entitled to our choices.

Life is what you make it. Take action. Choose happiness.

From there, we should approach each day of our lives by first being grateful for everything. When I started making that huge shift from expectation to gratitude, I felt the weight of the world come off my shoulders.

It helped me live in the moment. It helped me take time to smell the roses. It helped me be grateful for exactly what was happening—the good and the bad—in that moment. I became so enamored by the moment that I didn't have time to think about what was going to happen five days from now. I stopped expecting and demanding. I stopped focusing on how much I deserved.

We want for nothing and deserve nothing. Approach your life from a position of gratitude. Take the time to look at the beauty all around you, and be grateful for your opportunities. Be ever grateful for the miracle of this beautiful life.

Conclusion

In the world today, there are many challenges. So many people are struggling with conflicts in their personal lives, work, and health. Above all, what seems to be in shortest supply is hope.

Life is simple and we make it complicated. Life is hopeful in nature; it is not hopeless. If you can begin to think in a positive direction, you are going to attract more positivity, and more positivity is going to move your life in a different direction.

I am hoping that this book will offer something that will touch every reader's heart. Above all, I hope it helps to instill a new sense of hope.

The next step is to act.

Happiness is a choice and it demands action. In this book, I've given you some action steps to take to begin your journey. Remember, you don't always need to know where you are going; you just need to know if where you are is where you want to be. If this is not so, you've got to change your direction.

This isn't as hard as it may seem. If you don't like the direction in which your life is going, focus on changing one degree every day, just one degree. Think about it. If you change one degree every day, then in one hundred and eighty days, you are going to be going in the opposite direction.

One of my intentions was to make this book very short so that it serves as a pocket guide. We have so many books in our lives, and most of them we don't even read through. We're all busy, and our downtime is limited. Sometimes, after we have experienced something new—a book or a seminar—we finish it feeling inspired. This will last for a little while, but soon we find ourselves back to our old patterns. If you find this happening, then pick this book back up again. Or find another book. Don't be satisfied until you are happy.

Don't be satisfied with an unhappy life. Choose happiness. Choose action. Don't just sit there and do nothing. Don't just sit there thinking about it, keeping it in your head, keeping it to yourself. Talk about it with friends. If you have disagreements, talk about them. Take action.

All through this book, I have tried to share my own experiences, to tell you what got me through to the next level. I have shared the lessons I've learned about making life choices, about gratitude and patience.

Sometimes you are doing everything that you can for your life. You are making good choices, you are working hard on yourself and your relationships, and you are moving forward according to your life purpose. However, you still may not be feeling good.

In this case, remember that life has seasons, and sometimes, it's just wintertime. You batten down the hatches, and the snow piles up. You may feel more lethargic and face more depression during those gloomy days.

The point I am trying to make here is sometimes you must wait until springtime comes. Then the leaves come back on the trees, and the birds are singing again. You can get out in the fresh air where there is new life all around you. Sometimes, there's nothing more you need do at this moment than weather the storm and wait for better weather. And that's a lesson in patience.

I wish you a tremendous journey.

Next Steps

Visit our website to find more information about our practice and mission: docksidechiropractic.com

We are also on Facebook at: Dockside Chiropractic. Visit our page and *Like* us!

If you live in Brevard County, we invite you to contact us directly:

Dockside Chiropractic
1300 Pinetree Drive, Suite 7
Indian Harbour Beach, Florida 32937
321-775-3734

Mention this book and your initial consultation (value of $70) will be free!

About the Author

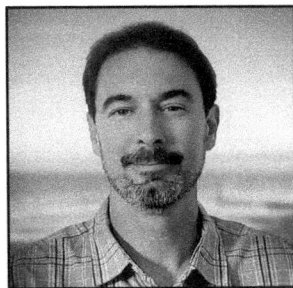

Dr. Kevin Poulston is a 2009 graduate of Life University College in Marietta, Georgia. While there, he served as Vice-President of the Conscious Chiropractic Club and was an active member of both the Chiropractic Philosophy Club and the Christian Chiropractic Club.

Kevin served as an ambassador to the Spinals Mission organization—an organization dedicated to bringing the chiropractic message to the countries of Central America through a series of mission trips and through the establishment of clinics throughout the region.

Dr. Poulston owns and practices energetic chiropractic care at Dockside Chiropractic, located in Indian Harbour Beach, Florida. His professional mission is help make Brevard County one of the healthiest, happiest communities in all of Florida through chiropractic.

www.ingramcontent.com/pod-product-compliance
Lightning Source LLC
Chambersburg PA
CBHW070759290326
41931CB00011BA/2083